The Top Superfoods for Weight Loss, Anti-Aging & Detox

by Neo Monefa

Table of Contents

1. Cacao
2. MACA
3. COCONUT OIL
4. ACAI
5. RAW APPLE CIDER VINEGER
6. AMERICAN BLUE BERRY
7. ELDERBERRY
8. MANUKA HONEY
9. MELATONIN
10. VITAMIN D3
11. ASTRAGALUS

12. CRACKED CHLORELLA
13. KOMBUCHA
14. ALMOND MILK vs DAIRY MILK
15. LEMON MYRTLE OIL
16. CINNAMON
17. BROCCOLI SPROUTS
18. GREEN TEA
19. HIMALAYAN SEA SALT
20. SOUR SOP
21. RED WINE
22. MUSHROOM
23. PROBIOTICS
24. KEFIR
25. TURMERIC ROOT
26. KALE
27. QUINOA
28. FLAXSEED

29. STEEL CUT OATS

30. THANK YOU FOR READING!

1. Cacao

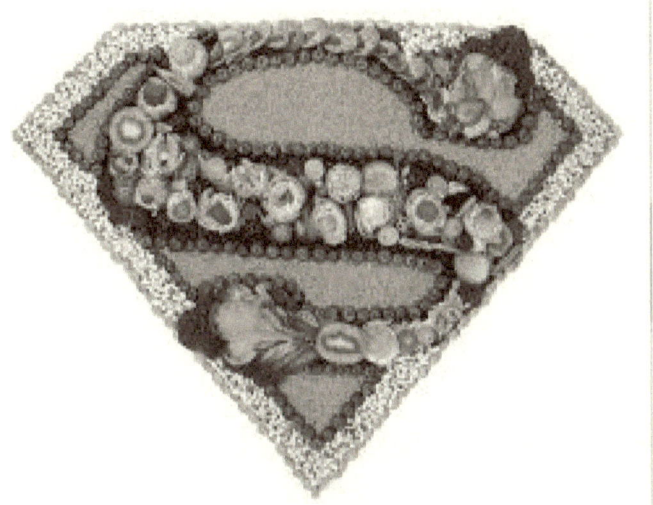

Theobroma Cacao

Cacao is a kind of bean from which the raw chocolate is produced and the tree from which the bean comes, is also called cacao. This evergreen tree is a tropical tree and cannot grow without the perfect temperature and condition. Cacao beans actually grow in the fruit, which is called cacao pods and the extracted beans are not only used as the source of cacao butter or chocolate but also these beans are similarly valuable to pharmaceutical use.

The history of cacao tree and use of the beans are foggy but it is believed that around 1500BC-400BBC the Olmec Indians in Mexico used to take a drink, which was made with the crushed cacao beans. Therefore it can be said that the Olmecs were the first people, who tasted chocolate. The Mayan people considered cacao as a divine fruit. Columbus was the first European, who tasted cacao but did not appreciate its taste. Finally it was reached to Spain and Portugal. Cacao has been introduced to United States as a form of chocolate by an Irish chocolate maker.

Therapeutic compositions in Cacao

In beans: Theobromine, Caffeine, Thiamine, Calcium, Riboflavin, Niacin, Calcium, Flavonols, Iron, Potassium, Magnesium, Fat, Amino Acids and Vitamins (A, C, D, E).

In butter: Stearic and palmitic acid, isoloic acid.

Medicinal use of cacao

Asthma: The chemical compound Theobromine in cacao helps to stop bronchospasms and also helps to open constricted bronchial passages. Theobromine relaxes the muscles inside throats and it opens the esophagus. So, taking cacao may help an asthma patient to take easier breath. In this way it also helps the patients, who are suffering from lung congestion, bronchitis,

High Blood Pressure: The antioxidant compound favonols, found in cacao and chocolate (especially in dark chocolate) contributes in formation of nitric oxide and thus opens up the blood vessels naturally. Dr Ried has shown that consuming cacao for the people with hypertensions could help to reduce blood pressure. Researcher of the National Institute of Integrative Medicine and the University of Adelaide in Australia says that flavanol-rich cocoa may "complement other treatment options and might contribute to reducing the risk of cardiovascular disease."

Other Medical benefits: Anandamide lipid in cacao helps to reduce the blood sugar level. Protein, fat, carbohydrate, zinc, iron magnesium and calcium are other beneficial compounds for health found in cacao and its products as well. Consuming cacao can help to form strong hair strong bones as it contains magnesium and high sulfur.

Controversial benefits: Some doctors have accepted that cacao can be the remedy for some health deformities, like- mall functioning of liver, stretch mark during pregnancy, kidney ailments, wrinkled skin, high cholesterol and diabetes. But many doctors reject this theory for insufficient evidences.

· Cacao is considered as the most addictive substance.

- It is a super toxic to liver.
- Much and regular consumption of raw cacao and chocolate may affect kidney.
- High amount of caffeine in cacao could be the cause of anxiety disorder.

Consuming huge amount of cacao or without medical super vision, it might be fatal for some patients suffering from – diarrhea, diabetes, IBS or GERD.

2. MACA

Lepidium Meyenii

Maca is a nutritious food with rich medicinal properties and this "Peruvian Ginseng" is praised as a natural Viagra in western world. Maca belongs to the potato family. We actually consume the powder of dried maca root, which is known as herbal supplement. From thousands of year people has been using maca for its natural ability to boost libido.

Record says, around 3800BC the Peruvian Inca people used to grow maca for extracting the nutritious and medicinal properties from the root. During the 16th century AD the Spanish people came to know about the herbal qualities of maca from the Inca people and brought it to Europe. In USA the scientists are engaged to discover other unknown medicinal benefits in maca.

Medicinal properties in Maca

Vitamins- B1, B2, B12, C, E; Minerals- zinc, iron, magnesium, calcium, phosphorus; amino acids, carbohydrates and number of glycosides.

Health benefits of Maca

Maca root has the biochemical functioning in human body. Scientists have shown that it has the capability to regulate the hormonal system, as it enhances the endocrine functions. Due to this capability maca powder consumption of maca can improve the fertility, sexual functions and digestion. According to the traditional medical theory maca also improves the nervous physiology and boosts the energy level.

Maca & Sex:

Maca has been praised since thousands of year for its effectiveness on male and female libido. A study Published in the Asian Journal of Andrology has shown that Maca increases libido. The research has shown that Maca dramatically improves the sex drive. It has been proven that the patients with mild erectile dysfunction can be treated with maca extracts. It is believed that maca is a herbal remedy for male impotence. It has been seen that the women who used to consume maca, got the increasing effect of having intercourse.

Researchers at Massachusetts General Hospital studied maca for its effect on selective serotonin reuptake inhibitor (SSRI) induced sexual dysfunction. They conducted a double-blind study comparing a low dose (1.5 g/day) to a high-dose (3.0 g/day) maca regimen in 20 depressed outpatients with SSRI induced sexual dysfunction. Patients receiving the higher dose showed a significant improvement on a sexual experience scale and sexual function questionnaire, while subjects on the lower dose did not. Libido improved significantly and was not differentiated by dose amount. Maca was well tolerated by both groups
(http://www.naturalnews.com/026413_maca_health_stress.html)

Other sexual Functions-
- It works as mood enhancement and energy booster.
- Maca is used for swollen prostate.
- It can be used as the treatment for menopause.
- It reduces menopause symptoms.
- Maca improves hormonal balance and testosterone level.
- It increases the production of sperms.
- It nourishes glandular system.

Other Health Benefits-

- **Balancing hormones:** Maca works on the pituitary gland to control the hormonal balance. Peruvian Maca root stimulates glands to produce the required hormones to restore the hormonal balance in body.
- **Reduces psychological symptoms in women:** The estrogenic and androgenic activity of maca can give the psychological stability to those women, who are going through postmenopausal period, without altering their hormone status.
- **Pain reliever:** Even a small amount of maca can alleviate pain.

- Maca is a source of natural fiber.
- It can prevent diabetes.
- Maca lowers the excessive blood pressure.

3. COCONUT OIL

Cocos Nucifera Oil

Coconut oil is an edible liquid that is extracted from the matured coconut kernel. This slightly sweet but nutty flavored oil has the wide variety of culinary uses as well as it contains some medical applications also.

Coconut has been used as a food and pharmaceutical for over 4000years. Around 1500BC, the Aryan civilization in India used this oil as a medicine related to mind, body and soul. The prolific use of coconut oil in tropical regions was being so respected. After the World War 2 coconut oil has been sold as coconut butter in USA.

Chemical Properties in Coconut Oil

* **Vitamin E & other organic particles.**
*__Fatty acid:__ coconut oil contains almost 94% of saturated fatty acids including a good percentage of medium-chain triglycerides.
*Saturated fats (medium chain) like Capric Acid, Caprylic Acid, Caproic Acid and Myristic Acid act as anti-oxidant.
*Other saturated fats- Palmitic acid, Stearic acid.
*Unsaturated fats - Linolenic acid, Linoleic acid and Oleic acid

Health Benefits of Coconut oil

Coconut oil has been praised worldwide from thousands of year for its medical values.
Traditional medicinal use of coconut oil: earache, fever, flu, gingivitis, gonorrhea, irregular or painful menstruation, asthma, baldness, bronchitis, bruises, burns, colds, tumors, typhoid, ulcers, upset stomach, weakness, and wounds.

Modern science also has discovered various pharmaceutical values in coconut oil.

Modern medicinal use of coconut oil: herpes, measles, hepatitis C, SARS, AIDS; kills parasites like tapeworms, lice, giardia; throat infections, urinary tract infections, gum disease, insulin secretion, cystic fibrosis, osteoporosis, periodontal, liver disease, kidney stones, inflammation.

Heart Disease: Many people have the misconception that consuming coconut oil may harm heart, as coconut oil contains large amount of saturated fats. But the actual fact is just opposite. The Medium Chain Triglycerides present in Coconut Oil lowers the level of bad cholesterol and lowers the risk of having heart attack. Lauric acid prevents high blood pressure as well as coconut oil helps to prevent atherosclerosis.

Weight Loss: The medium chain fatty acids helps to improve the functions of thyroid and endocrine system. Coconut oil gradually increases the metabolic rate in human body and thus it helps to burn more energy or fats. Finally it comes as a result of weight loss. So, consuming coconut oil regularly prevents obesity.

Immunity: The anti-microbial lipids, lauric acid, capric acid and caprylic in coconut oil help to strengthen the immunity system due to their anti-fungal, antibacterial and antiviral properties. Even, some Doctors believe that coconut oil contains the properties to fight against HIV.

Other Medicinal Uses
- It can be used as brain boosting, head lice-clearing, wounds-healing.
- Improves digestive disorders.
- Reduces the chance of having cancer.
- Protects the skins from having cracks.
- Fights against candida.
- Acts as testosterone booster.
- Improves blood lipids.

4. ACAI

Euterpe Oleracea

Acai is a berry fruit, which comes from the acai palm mostly found in the Amazon estuary. The amazing thing is that the seed of this fruit acquires almost 90% of the total fruit and only the skin is edible. Usually acai is used for making juice and some desserts as well as delicious sorbets. The powder, made with dried acai is sometimes added to many foods and it contains high anti-oxidant.

More than four thousand years old history of acai tells that the Amazon people first discovered the medical values in acai and they used to take it to get rid of various ailments. Acai fruit has been used as natural anti-oxidant and natural cholesterol controller. The Amazon tribes also knew that acai berry could help to build immune system, protect heart and fights against prostate diseases. Acai was introduced globally after 1980.

Chemical Composition in Acai Berr

Anti-Oxidant: Anthocyanins(polyphenolic anthocyanin - cyanidin-3 –galactoside, resveratrol, petunidin, delphinidin), Flavonoids, Phenols, Proanthocyanidins and Xanthones.
Vitamins: A, B1, B2, B3, C, E and K.
Minerals: Phosphorus, Iron, Calcium, Potassium, Magnesium, Zinc and Copper.
Omegas: Omega3, Omega6 and Omega9.

Health Benefits of Acai

With the rich amount of Anthocyanins, acai berry acts as anti-inflammatory and anti-cancer agent. Scientists say that acai fruit is the source of highest nutritional supply and it gives our body some important nutritional elements that cannot be typically found in regular diet. Due to its large medical properties acai berries can be available in health grocers too.

Heart and Cholesterol: Omega6 and Omega9 fatty acids help to protect the entire cardiovascular system and control the heart health as well as these fatty acids help to lower the cholesterol level. The adequate dietary fiber in acai helps to clear cholesterol through stools.
Weight Loss: It organically increases the metabolism rate in body and thus more calories need to be burnt. So, regular consumption of acai would help to prevent obesity.

Anti-oxidant: Anti-oxidant property plays the most important role in the therapeutic use of acai berry. It helps to prevent free radicals and removes toxins from body, as well as can help repairing cell damages.

Other Therapeutic Uses:
· Controls digestive health.
· Increases stamina.
· Amino acids and monounsaturated essential oils and minerals help to improve arterial health.

- Studies suggest that Ellagic acid in acai fruit can directly inhibit DNA binding carcinogens.
- In traditional medicine, acai has been used as medicine to treat parasitic infections, hemorrhages and diarrhea. Acai powder was believed to be the remedy for fever.

5. RAW APPLE CIDER VINEGER

Catabolic Fermented Food

Raw cider vinegar has been used for over centuries not only just for the culinary benefits but also as folk remedies. It has been called "natural miracle", as it has the ability to treat many ailments. Record says that Chinese people knew the benefits of this vinegar from as early as 1500BC. According to ancient Assyrian writings natural apple cider vinegar was used to treat earache. Even in Bible, apple cider vinegar was recorded as an antiseptic and healing agent. In USA it is not added with alcohol.

The commercially produced ACV should be avoided, as the pasteurization and filtration during the process of making ACV destroy and remove the "Mother", which is considered to be beneficial to health. So, you should consume the traditional apple cider vinegar and the always prefer to use the ACV made from perfect and healthy apples.

Beneficial Ingredients

- · Acetic acid.
- · Raw Enzymes.
- · Vitamins – A, B1, B2, B6, C, E, P and Provitamin beta-carotene.
- · Minerals- Iron, Copper, Sulfur, Sodium, Magnesium, Potassium and Chlorine Phosphorous.

Health Benefits of unfiltered Raw ACV

- · It can treat colds and flue.

- Reduces sore throats and sinus infection.
- Medicine for- **Constipation, Diarrhea, Gas** or **Indigestion.**
- **Can fight against infection.**
- **It lowers blood pressure and controls cholesterol.**
- **Rich amount of calcium in ACV promote strong bones and teeth.**
- **ACV can be useful to prevent heart disease.**
- **External uses to treat- age spots, ear infection, nosebleeds, vaginal yeast infection and Eczema.**
- Regular use of raw ACV can reduce weights, as it breaks the fats and prevents storing fats in body.
- Raw ACV can inhibit cancer cells and slower their growth.

Mother: Most of the commercially produced ACVs lack this important ingredient during the filtration. Only raw organic and unfiltered apple cider vinegar contains "mother' and appears to be most potent remedies. Mother is a naturally occurring enzyme, which is a composition of composition of protein molecules, nutrients and beneficial bacteria.

6. AMERICAN BLUE BERRY

Vaccinium Corymbosum

3500 years old colorful history describes that the Native American people used dried blue berries in soups and used to add the powdered blue berries into meat as preservative. Native Americans gathered the wild blue berries that grew in North America and used the berries, leaves, and roots for medicinal purposes. Surprisingly blue berry remained an uncultivated fruit before early 20th century. In early 1900's the pioneered botanist at the United States Department of Agriculture, Dr. Fredrick Coville first introduced the cultivation process of blue berry with the help of Elizabeth White, who established the first commercial blueberry field.

Chemical Compounds
·   Protein.
·   Vitamins- A, B1, B2, C, E and P.
·   Mineral- Phosphorus, Calcium.
·   Excellent Source of phytochemicals.
·   Anthocyanins.
·   Phenolics.
·   Flavonoid antioxidants- carotene-β, lutein and Zea-xanthin
·   Proanthocyanidins

Health Benefits
The Anthocyanins in blueberry is believed to have health benefits and plays the role as an antioxidant. Anthocyanins are the only fatty acids that can improve night vision, reduces the risk of having heart disease.

- Blueberries are among the fruits that contain highest rate of natural antioxidant compounds.
- The phyto-chemicals compounds protect our body from free radicals and thus it helps to prevent cancer and degenerative diseases.
- Vitamin B-6, niacin, riboflavin, pantothenic acid and folic acid help our body to metabolize fat, carbohydrates and proteins.

Eye Care: It is believed that due to vitamin A and other compounds blueberry is able to prevent age related ocular problems like cataracts, myopia, hypermetropia, macular degeneration and retina infection. The anti oxidant carotenoids along with selenium, zinc and vitamin A, C and E are very essential for eye health.

Cancer: Anthocyanins, Proanthocyanidins, flavonols and tannins in blue berries can inhibit the cancer cells and restrict their growth. Researches have shown that regular eating of blue berries is very much beneficial to prevent colon cancer and ovarian cancer.

Brain Health: Some recent studies have shown that eating blue berries is good for memory function and maintaining brain health. All the antioxidant properties and minerals can heal neurotic disorders as well as prevent degeneration of neurons. These properties can even heal the damaged brain cells and keep the memory sharp. It is also believed that to the some extent blue berry is very helpful to cure Alzheimer's.

Immunity: Blueberries are rich in antioxidants, vitamins (C, E, B complex), copper along with other anti bacterial substances, which are very effective to build body immunity.

Other health Benefits: prevents constipation and improves digestion, prevents heart disease, can be used as antidepressant, helps to cure Urinary Tract infection, reduces cholesterol, acts an anti-aging.

Traditional Therapeutic Use:
- Hemorrhoids.
- Glaucoma.

- Sore throats.
- Diarrhea.
- Appetite stimulation.
- Urinary tract infection.

7. ELDERBERRY

Sambucus Nigra

Elderberry has been used as herbal fruit from the historical periods. Though elderberry is native to Europe and Asia but it has wide spread in USA also. This fruit is also a staple supply of foods for many birds. During the spring time it blooms as aromatic white flowers and then it is called elderflowers. Elderflower is not only used to make jellies but it is brewed into wines and champagne also. Among the several varieties of elderberry, the purple berries are the most plentiful. But be careful about the fact that all the parts of the elderberry tree are not edible as they contain toxin. Only the ripe blossoms and fruits can be safely used as food or medicine.

Chemical Compounds in Elderberry fruits

- Phenolics, including kaempferol, rutin, quercetin and phenolic acids.
- Anthocyanins.
- Vitamins- A & C.

So, it can be said that elderberry fruits are the excellent source of antioxidants, vitamins and important minerals such as iron and calcium. Along with these components, these fruits also contain some essential oils, tannins and sterols to be a healthy food.

Health Benefits

- It has been proven that elderberry can fights against eight different influenzas. It is also verymuch effective against H1N1 viral infection.
- Studies have shown that cinnamon in elderberry prevent HIV to from infecting target cells.
- Elderberry boosts the immunity system.
- It is helpful to reduce weights.
-

One should always take advice from doctor before taking elderberry extracts or syrup to know the optimal dosage and to avoid drug interactions. Though elderberry fruits and other parts of this tree are not recommended for raw use, as these are very much toxic but only the sambucus nigra is the only variety, which is non-toxic.

8. MANUKA HONEY

Monofloral Honey

Manuka honey has been treated as the must have medicine to be applied on wounds as well as the natural sweetener in drinks since long periods. The aboriginal people in New Zealand have used this honey for centuries. This mono-floral honey is made by the bees collecting pollen from the Leptospermum Scoparium tea flowers in New Zealand. The ancient people knew that the natural properties in honey could be the remedy of many ailments.

Medicinal properties in Manuka Honey

Hydrogen peroxide- it gives the anti biotic quality.
Methylglyoxal- anti-bacterial.
Glucose Oxidase enzyme – it slowly releases hydrogen peroxide.
The UMF (Unique Manuka Factor) scale rates the potency of Manuka honey and it corresponds with the concentration of mythylglyoxal.

Health Benefits

The anti bacterial properties along with other unique compounds make manuka honey beneficial for health. Medical studies have shown that manuka honey is not only beneficial for its anti-bacterial properties but also it is a potent anti-oxidant. Anicient people used to appli it on the wounds and dressing for burn to prevent infection.

Here is a list of medical use of manuka honey-
- This honey has the anti-inflamation properties.
- It prevents infection by destroying bacteria.
- It hastens the healing process.
- Manuka honey cures ringworm and other fungal conditions.
- It fights against antibiotic-resistant strains of bacteria (MRSA & VRE).
- Studies have shown it is useful to treat diabetes.
- It can cure gastrointestinal problems.
- Active manuka honey lowers the level of cholesterol.

· Even it can be used as the remedy for eye, ear and sinus infection.

9. MELATONIN

N-acetyl-5-methoxytryptamine

This natural occurring hormone is found in humans, animals, plants and microbes. Melatonin controls the sleep regulations and is made in the pineal gland, which is a pea size gland structured at the center of the brain. Melatonin can also be found in stomach and intestines. Melatonin also influences the activities of some other hormones in body.

Functions of Melatonin in our body

Melatonin controls the circadian rhythm, which is actually our body's own internal clock. It decides when to fall asleep and when to wake up. The secretion of this hormone depends on how the dark or light our surroundings are. The light sensitive receptors in our eyes relay the report of surroundings conditions to suprachiasmatic nucleus situated in our brain and then suprachiasmatic nucleus orders the pineal gland to secrete or stop producing melatonin. When it is dark in outside melatonin is being produced more and when it is light the production drops. That is why we fall asleep at night and wake up in the morning naturally. If the conditions of the surrounding are changed forcefully or if we go against the internal clock, the regulation of melatonin got broken and disrupted and it may be the cause of cancer. Studies show that the people, who work night shifts regularly, may be at the high risk of having cancer.

Melatonin also controls the frequency and duration menstrual cycles in woman body, as it regulates the production of women's reproductive hormones. That is why melatonin is responsible for menopause.

The level of melatonin is related to our age. Studies describe that the level of melatonin drops, as we grow older. That is why children have the highest level of melatonin.

It is believed that the disruption of melatonin level in women body may the fatal cause of having breast cancer. Actually the women suffering from breast cancer tend to have lower level of melatonin than the normal women have.

Being a strong anti oxidant melatonin may strengthen the immune system in our body.

Foods that contain Melatonin

The Journal of Pineal Research have studied that the melatonin rich foods contain very lower amount than the supplements doses have but able to increase the level of melatonin in blood.

"According to the Society for Light Treatment and Biological Rhythms, approximately 5-25 mcg of melatonin circulate in the blood stream of healthy young and middle-aged men at night time. If we take an average of 15 mcg, which equals 15,000 ng this number can serve us as a comparison to foods with melatonin" (source-http://www.thehealersjournal.com/2013/04/08/foods-high-in-melatonin)

Amount of melatonin in some foods:
- Cherries – Cherries are the only natural food to supply highest amount of melatonin.
- Banana- Banana contains L-tryptophan (amino acid), which is converted into 5-HTP in brain and this 5-HTP turns into melatonin and serotonin.
- Cherry juice- 17,535 ng/gm
- Mustard seeds- 191.33 ng/gm
- Peanuts- 116.70 ng/gm
- Corn – 187.80 ng/gm
- Rice- 149.80 ng/gm
- Barley grains- 87.30 ng/gm
- Rolled oats – 79.13 ng/gm

Is Melatonin Suppliments safe?

Some research suggests that melatonin supplements may be helpful to treat -

- Insomnia
- Jet lag,
- Seasonal affective disorders,
- To control the sleep patterns for those people who work night shift.
- Chronic cluster headache.
- To slow down the growth of cancer.
- To make the immune system stronger.

But those supplements come with some side effects like –

- Daytime Sleepiness
- Headaches.
- Dizziness.
- Lower body temperature.
- Changes in blood pressure.
- Mild anxiety.
- Abdominal discomfort.

These supplements may interact with some medications like –

- Diabetes
- Birth control pills.
- Anticoagulants

Before taking supplements melatonin, one must take advice from specialized doctor. Meltanonin should be given to children and pregnant women under doctor supervision.#

10. VITAMIN D3

Cholecalcifero

Fat-soluble secosteroids (vitamin D) enhance the intestinal absorption of calcium and phosphate in our body and vitamin D3 plays the most important role in this secosteroids. Deficiency in vitamin D3 is still an epidemic in this advanced medical era. Some recent studies have reviewed that the main cause of vitamin D3 deficiency in USA is due to the lack of exposure to sunlight.

Vitamin D3 is not only a vitamin but also it acts as a hormone. The vitamin D3 (as a hormone) controls phosphorus, and bone metabolism as well as neuro- muscular functions. Calcium cannot be digested in human body without adequate amount of Vitamin D3.

Forms of Vitamin D3:

- **Cholecalciferol -** Unhydroxylated form of vitamin D3.
- **Calcifediol** – *hydroxycholecalciferol, also known as 25-hydroxyvitamin D3.*
- **Calcitriol- The active form of vitamin D3,**

Vitamin D3 Deficiency

Ricket: This is a kind of childhood disease, which is characterized by soft, weak, impeded growth and deformity of bone. Lack of vitamin D3 is the main reason for this disease.

Osteoporosis: This disease decreases the mineral density in bones and thus small holes appear in the bones.

Osteomalacia: Due to the deficiency of Vitamin D, adult people may fall into this disease, in which the bones become soften and cause of proximal muscle weakness.

Skin Pigmentation: The lack of vitamin D3 synthesis from sun may be the cause of pigmentation.

Other disease –

· Obesity
· High
· Blood pressure,
· Type2 diabetes
· Chronic fatigue syndrome
· Kidney stones
· Depression
· Fibromalgia
· Alzheimer's
· Even leads to have breast, prostate and colon cancer

Benefits of Vitamin D3

· **Bone Health:** Vitamin D3 plays an important role to improve bone health and musculoskeletal system. D3 can act to regulate the mechanisms of parathyroid hormone (PTH) and decreases secondary hyperparathyroidism.
· **Cancer:** Studies have proven that who has the potential amount of D3, is having the lesser risk to have cancer.
· **Alzheimer's:** It reduces the chance of having Alzheimer's.
· **It maintains the mental health.**
· **Vitamin D3 reduces the back pain.**
· **This vitamin has the ability to improve cognition.**
· **Immunity:** Vitamin D3 regulates the T cells and this T cells have an important role to improve immune system in our body. Vitamin D3 prevents the excessive expression of inflammatory cytokines and increases the efficiency of macrophages. Vitamin D3 protects our lungs from infection by stimulating peptides.

Vitamin D3 Excess

Regular large doses of vitamin D3 may increase the level of this vitamin in our body and may be the cause of some malfunctions of body organs or factors. Excessive Vitamin D3 can develop the toxic accumulation of the nutrient.

Some worst effects of vitamin D3 efficiency:

- Kidney problems.
- Bone Loss.
- Cardiovascular problems.

Sources of Vitamin D3

The main source of D3 is exposure of skins to the Sun. In Sunlight our skin synthesizes Vitamin D3. At least 15 minutes daily under the sun can be enough to fulfill the minimum requirement of D3 in our body.

Food Sources:

- **Fish:** Raw fatty fish contains more vitamin D than the cooked one. Raw Atlantic Herrings contains 1628IU per 100grams. Other fishes – Oil packed Tuna, Oil packed Saradines, Canned Salmon and Raw Mackerel etc.
- **Cord liver Oil:** Cord liver oil has been considered as the best supplement for vitamin D3, as it contains 10001IU/100grams vitamin D3.
- **Oysters:** This is the other great source other than cord liver oil.
- **Fortified Products:** Most tofu and cereals are fortified with vitamin. Soy products- Silk light soymilk, soy yogurt.
- **Fortified Dairy Products:** Milk- 52.0IU/100grams, Cheese- 6.6IU/100grams,
- **Black & Red Caviar.**
- **Eggs- 37.0IU/ 100grams and fried egg - 17.0IU.**
- **Mushrooms- 27.0IU/100grams.**

There are also various Vitamin D supplements available in market but no one should take those without medical supervision and may cautious about the side effects.

11. ASTRAGALUS

Astragalus Membranaceus

Astragalus has been considered as a renowned medicine in Traditional Chinese Medicine for thousand of years. Ancient Chinese people believed that astragalus could stimulate the immune system and strengthen the digestion. It was often combined with other herbs to increase the immunity power in body.

The medical name of astragalus is *Astragalus membranaceus. It is also known as* huang ch', bei qi, radix astragali, green dragon and milk vetch root etc. Astragalus belongs to the Leguminosae plant family. Astragalus actually a type of bean and the root of this plant is used as medicine. There are more than 2000 species available worldwide but the medical varieties grow only in western and central Asia. There are two very similar verities used for medical purpose- Astragalus membranaceus mongholicus and Astragalus membranaceus leguminosae.

Medicinal properties

Triterpenoid saponins:

- **Astragenol**
- Acetylastragalosides I-X
- Alosistragades I – VIII
- Isoastragalosides I-IV
- Soyasaponin I

Amino Acids:

- GABA
- l-canavanine

Other compounds:

- Isoflavonoids - calycosin and formononetin
- Cycloastragenol 6
- 25-di-O-beta-D-glucopyranoside
- Polysaccharides - astragalan, astraglucan AMem-P
- Selenium
- Volatile oil
- Plant sterols

Medicinal Use

* The root of this plant contains the medicinal properties and this root is used for both medicinal and culinary purposes.

Astragalus root is an immune-stimulant, pectoral, anti-inflammatory, antiviral, Cardio-tonic, diuretic, anhydrotic (stops sweating), anti-hypertensive, antibacterial and adaptogen.
Research, held in USA has shown that astragalus can be the possible treatment for those, whose immune system got weakened by chemotherapy. Being an anti-oxidant it can be the remedy for heart disease. Astragalus root is often used as an ingredient of tonic wine and tea.

- The patients, who are going through chemotherapy can take astragalus to prevent farther liver damage due to the radiation.
- It helps to grow the natural resistance, so, it can be a possible treatment for cold and flu.
- It delivers the diuretic effect and thus it lowers the blood pressure.
- Astragalus helps to stimulate body to produce interferon for defending against viral infections.
- By nourishing exhausted adrenals it fights against fatigue.

- Astragalus has anti-bacterial and anti-inflammatory properties and so, it can be applied on wounds to prevent infection.
- Due to the richness in Polysaccharides, it supports the overall immune system.
- Astragalus contains the anti-clotting and vaso-dialating. That is why it prevents coronary heart disease.
- According to a study held in China, it improves sperm motility.
- This herb fights against the formation of kidney stone.
- Astragalus also fights against Proteusbacteria and prevents bladder infections.

12. CRACKED CHLORELLA

A Nutrient-Rich Algae

Chlorella has been found as an individual whole food dietary supplement. Single-celled fresh-water algae, chlorella is among the most ancient life forms on the earth and is virtually unchanged in over 2 billion years of existence. Thus, it harbors the spark that characterized the original creative energy of the planet (http://www.naturodoc.com/chlorella.htm).

It is believed that the cell wall surrounding the chlorella is indigestible, so the cell needs to be broken in order to get the benefits of its nutrients.

Chemical Compounds

Therapeutic agents:

Amino acids – Lysine, Cystine, Histidine, Arginine, Methionine, Aspartic acid, Threonine, Glutamic acid, Phenylalanine, Glycine and others.

Vitamins - A, B1, B2, B6, C and E

Minerals - Iron, Zinc, Copper, Calcium, Magnesium and Phosphorus.

Saturated and Unsaturated fatty acids,

Nutrients:

Lipids, Carbohydrates, Proteins and food fibers.

Highly concentrated components:

Chlorophyll, Chlorellin, Sporopollein and Chlorella Growth Factor.

Health Benefits

Studies have claimed that chlorella is able to fight against cancer, bacterial and viral infections due to its anti oxidant properties. It has also shown that cracked chlorella increases the level of albumin to maintain a good blood health. A study held in 1960 claimed that chlorella decreases the side effects of chemotherapy. In Japan it is popularly consumed to protect the body from the history old nuclear radiation.

Benefits of the compounds

Chlorophyll:
- Prevents the growth of kidney stones.
- Helps to stabilize blood pressure.
- Maintains heart health by fortifying heart muscle.
- It inhibits the harmful free radicals.
- Improves intestinal transit.
- Heals the wounds.
- It also act as detoxifier.

Sporopollein: This compound actually acts as a detoxifier and thus it frees our body from the toxic components like heavy metals and organic solvents. Use of chlorella is a traditional method to remove toxins from human body.

Chlorellin: Due to this compound, chlorella is called natural antibiotic. Chlorella works on the one hand like a probiotic, by favouring the growth and diffusion of natural acido-lactic bacteria in the vagina or in the large intestines.

CGF (Chlorella Growth Factor)
- It helps to increase the natural resistance in our body.

- It works as a booster to immunity system.
- Diabetes patient can be treated with chlorella as it contains CGF.
- The nucleic acid in CGF prevents the continual weakening of immune system.

Other Therapeutic Use:

Withdrawals from drug addiction, Alcohol hangover prevention, cholesterol, high blood pressure, atherosclerosis, pancreatitis, peptic ulcers, duodenal ulcers, gastritis (9), diabetes, heart disease, cancer,anti-viralgout,arthritis, allergies, anemia, asthma, cold, cold sores, flu, bad breath, body odors, acne and skin problems, burns, wound healing,

13. KOMBUCHA

Red Tea Mushroom

Sugary black tea is fermented with the help of SCOBY (symbiotic culture of bacteria and yeast) to produce the healthy carbonated drink "Kombucha". Some people say that it tastes like the combination of champagne and apple cider but actually the taste depends upon what kind of tea is being used. Kombucha contains the probiotic benefits with the refreshing aroma.

The records and evidences depict that kombucha originated in Tsin Dunasty (about 220BC) in ancient china and they praise it as "the tea of immortality". Some historical events also show that in 12th century Genghis Khan and his army used to drink kombucha for the strength and vitality. It then traveled to Russia and there it was taken as an effective folk medicine in many rural communities and they called it Cajnyj Kvas. Soon it got its way to Japan and India. In 414 AD Dr. Kombu from Korea brought it to Japan to treat Japanese emperor Inkyo. In United States of America Kombucha has gained its popularity as a healthy beverage since the last 2 or 3 decades.

Chemical Comounds in Kombucha

- **Organic Acids: Glucuronic Acid, Lactic Acid, Acetic Acid, Usnic Acid, Oxalic Acid, Malic acid, Gluconic Acid, Butyric acid, Usnic Acid.**
- **Vitamins:** B1, B2, B3, B6 and C.
- **Amino Acid**
- **Folic Acid**
- **Antiseptic, Antibiotic and detoxifying characteristics.**

Health Benefits

After World War-II, the Russian researchers found that instead of higher tobacco and alcohol consumption level, two particular regions in the country were almost cancer free, and farther research have shown that the people of those two regions used to drink large amount of kombucha as habit. These Russian research perhaps the first modern scientific evidence that Kombucha is a body detoxifier and immune system booster. It has been also noticed in Japan that the women, who used to consume Kombucha regularly were free from wrinkles and other virtual signs of aging.

Benefits of organic acids-

- **Butyric acid: It protects human cellular membranes and fights against yeast infection.**
- **Oxalic Acid: It stimulates the intercellular production of energy.**
- **Gluconic Acid: It can be a great treatment for thrush infection.**
- **Acetic Acid: It inhibits some harmful bacteria.**
- **Usnic Acid: It acts as a natural antibiotic.**
- **Lactic Acid: It helps to regulate blood pH level and improves the digestive system.**
- **Glucuronic acid: This is the most important organic acid that acts as a detoxifier.**

Therapeutic Use-

Antibiotic: The antibiotic properties, primarily from the usnic acid, only develop after the 7th or 8th day. They also require a brewing temperature above 23C. The acetic acid bacteria produced are strongly antagonistic to streptococci, diplococci, flexner and shigella.

Detoxification: Being a detoxifier kombucha helps to have healty liver and aides cancer prevention. Kobucha contains many organic acids and enzymes, which detox our body and thus reduce the pancreatic load.

Joint care and skin care: Glucosamines in kombucha can prevent and even can treat all forms of arthritis. "Glucosamines increase synovial hyaluronic acid production. Hyaluronic acid functions physiologically to aid preservation of cartilage structure and prevent arthritic pain, with relief comparable to NSAIDs and advantage over glucocorticoids. Hyaluronic acid enables connective tissue to bind moisture thousands of times its weight and maintains tissue structure, moisture, lubrication and flexibility and lessens free radical damage, while associated collagen retards and reduces wrinkles (http://www.foodrenegade.com/kombucha-health-benefits/).

Other Therapeutic uses- Improves blood quality, it balances acidity, it increases stamina and energy, improves and maintains mental health and kombucha is a great immune booster.

14. ALMOND MILK vs DAIRY MILK

The milk from natural plant sources like nut, grains or soy is quickly acquiring the place of the dairy sources. Though they are gone through different procedures during processing and differ from each other regarding the containing components. "Which is better or healthier?"- this is the question, which always lingers into our mind whenever we come to a super market to buy a packet of milk. Among the natural plant sources, almond occupies an important role. So, here we will try to drag the better one by comparing their medicinal components and their therapeutic benefits.

ALMOND MILK

Almond milk has been used as the substitute of dairy milk from the medieval period. Finely ground almond is mixed with water t produce almond milk and this substitute milk has been a popular beverage in medieval Europe, as well as in the Middle East. It was also more acceptable than the dairy milk, as it had a long self-life. It travelled to USA with the European immigrants and soon it has found its popular place as alternative milk in USA households. The finer blended almond results a finer consistency of milk and the modern blending technology makes this option much easier. Some people think that the cooked foods contain the deprived amount of minerals or vitamins, where as the raw food is believed to be higher in nutrients. Almond milk has easily become popular to them.

Naturally made almond milk is sugar free and low in cholesterol but there are some flavored almond milk also available in market and this flavored alternative milk is high in added sugar. So, raw almond milk is always recommended.

Nutrition Facts

Calcium: Calcium is an essential mineral that strengthens our bones but in our body it is among the most abandoned thing by mass. So, fulfilling the necessity of calcium is must and therefore we should include foods containing calcium in daily diets. Like other milks, almond milk is also a source of calcium and 1cup of almond milk contains about 200mg of calcium.

Potassium & Sodium: 1cup of almond milk contains about 180mg potassium and 150mg sodium. Deficiency of potassium in our body may be the cause of many cardiac dysfunctions and on the other hand sodium produces cell membrane charges, which is necessary for the transmission of nerve impulses.

Protein: Protein does many important tasks in our body, including maintaining the body and its growth, utilizing membranes, forming blood cells, and being precursors to different bodily fluids, hormones, and molecules. Almond milk can be a source of protein though 1cup of almond milk contains about 1gram protein (less than dairy milk).

Saturated and Unsaturated Fat Content: Almond milk is beneficial to reduce the heart disease as it is a source of unsaturated fats. The healthy thing is that almond milk does not contain any of cholesterol and saturated fats.

Other Vitamins & Minerals:
- Vitamin E- it helps to slow down aging.
- Magnesium – It assists the functioning of the parathyroid glands.
- Manganese – It helps to activate the role of various enzymes in our body.
- Selenium – It increases the immune level.
- Vitamin A

Flavonoid and Antioxidant: The skin of almond is rich in flavonoids. So the almond always should be crushed with the skin. Almond milk is also contains anti-oxidants properties, so, it is also beneficial to prevent cancer.

Sugar or Carbohydrate: Almond milk does not contain sugar as well as it contains very lower amount of carbohydrate. So, drinking homemade almond is safe for diabetes patients.

Health Benefits

- **Heart Health:** Almond milk helps us to maintain better heart health, as it contains no cholesterol and very lower amount of sodium. The potassium in almond milk also helps to maintain normal and healthy blood pressure.
- **Weight loss:** Home-made almond milk has very lower amount of calories. Thus, it does not indulge to store extra calories in our body.
- **Eye Health:** Almond milk contains a moderate level of vitamin A, so, it is helpful for our eye health.
- **Lactose free-** Some people cannot take lactose because it would be the cause abdominal discomfort and diarrhea. Almond milk serves an important health benefits to them, as it is completely lactose free.
- **Other health benefits-** blood sugar friendly, improves bone health, can be used as skin care and gives more muscle power.

http://almondmilk.net/almond-milk-nutrition/

Almond Milk Vs Dairy Milk

- **Chemical Contamination**

Dairy milks tend to concentrate chemical compounds as hormones are injected and various chemical mixed foods are served to generate more milk. Small amount of toxins can be found in dairy milk. Dairy milk may be the cause of hormone imbalance or toxic effects in human body.

Almond milk is produced from the natural almond nuts so drinking almond milk is safe. Milk made from pesticides almond also has less contamination from chemicals.

Cholesterol fact

Dairy Milk and almond milk both are low in containing cholesterol.

Always keep in mind that excessively low and excessively high cholesterol both are dangerous for health.

Antibiotics and growth hormones

Detectable levels of antibiotics and growth hormones can be found in dairy milks. The antibiotics may be the cause of allergic reactions and other side effects for some people and it will make our body antibiotic resistant, which is a global health problem. A Harvard University research study indicates that the growth hormones increase the risk of having certain types of cancer in human body.

Regarding this fact Almond milk is safer to intake.

Sugar and protein facts

Home-made almond milk contains no sugar unlike dairy milk and that is why it is helpful for the diabetes patients.

On the other hand almond milk has much lesser amount of protein than dairy milk. So, almond milk cannot be a better source of protein than dairy milk.

Lactose

Dairy milk contains a large numbers of lactose, which can be the cause of allergy to some people. That is why some people turn their face far from dairy milks. Almond milk is the best alternative for those, who are suffering from casein or gluten allergy, as almond milk is completely lactose free.

· **Vitamin B factor**
This is one of the major differences between almond milk and dairy milk. Dairy milk contains more Vitamin B12 as well as riboflavin than almond milk.

· **Nutritional value**
The high level calcium in dairy milk is fortified with vitamin A and D to fulfill the regular requirements of these vitamins in our body. But almond milk contains wide range of necessary vitamins and that is why almond milk obtains the higher nutritional value than dairy milk.

· **Health Value**
Many people cannot consume dairy milks since it contains lactose and naturally occurring sugar. A large number of people cannot have the tolerance to lactose. However, dairy milk supplies the required protein to our body but almond milk does not.
In comparison to dairy milk, almond milk is much healthier food to be consumed. Almond milk is the wide source of vitamins and minerals. Almond milk contains some anti-oxidant properties; therefore it can combat against cancer.

· **Preservation**
Preservation is the major concern for every household. Dairy milk cannot be preserved for long time (not more than 3 days),

whereas, almond milk can last for long. Else, the nut almond can be preserved for a long time and whenever needed it can be ground and mixed with water.

15. LEMON MYRTLE OIL

Backhousia Citriodora (Oil)

Lemon Myrtle oil comes from the leaves of the tree Backhousie Citriodora, named after the English botanist Backhousia. Lemon Myrtle generally grows in the rainforest in Australia. The oil from it has been praised for its germicidal powers and has been used as Aromatherapy for long years. Discovery of the medicinal properties in lemon myrtle is not more than half a century long. A German company, Schimmel & Co made the first distillation of lemon Myrtle and after some years the Imperial Institute of London analyzed the lemon myrtle oil to introduce the medicinal properties in it. This oil has the distinct strong aroma of lemon due to the citral substance. The complex green note of this oil gives more depth in lemon aroma and staying power. It has been enriching the culinary, cosmetic and pharmaceutical industries for years.

Chemical Properties
Major Lemon Myrtle essential oil components analyzed through by Gas Chromatography

- B-Myrcene
- 6-methyl-5hepten-2-one
- Linalool
- Citronellal
- Cis-Isocitral
- Trans-Isocitra
- Nerol
- Cis-Isogeraniol
- Neral
- Eugenol
- Neryl Acetate

- Geranial
- Geraniol

This complex and composite oil contains over 50different chemical compounds. Citrals is the most dominant constituents of this oil.
"Citral is an aliphatic aldehyde in the monoterpenoid class. In plants such as lemongrass (Cymbopogon) and lemon balm (Melissa officinalis), citral occurs as two isomeric aldehydes, neral and geranial. Relative density: 0.89, refractive index 1.4928, optical rotation 1.0, solubility in 70% v/v ethanol 20 degrees C: 1.5ml" (http://www.uncleharrys.com/blog/product-library/post/lemon-myrtle-oil).

Health Benefits

Studies have shown that lemon myrtle oil contains antiseptic, analgesic, anti-rheumatic, expectorant, astringent, anti-neuralgic and anticonvulsant properties. Being a big source of anti-oxidant properties it has wide variety of therapeutic uses. According to Encyclopedia of Natural Medicine lemon myrtle oil can be used to treat common cold, influenza, raw throat, bronchitis, fatigue, sinus infections, allergies, dental infections, itching and athletes foot. Lemon myrtle scores a 16 on the Rideal-Walker scale and thus it is a potent anti-microbial.

The key ingredient in lemon myrtle oil is the high concentration of citral, which is a powerful anti-oxidant, non-acidic and anti-fungal agent.

According to "Therapeutic Herb Manual " lemon myrtle oil fights against various types of bacteria, such as Pseudomonas aeruginosa and Clostridium perfringens. It inhibits Helicobacter pylori bacteria to prevent gastrointestinal disorders. Other studies demonstrate that this oil is also helpful to reduce cellulite and it helps to strengthen the immune system as well.

16. CINNAMON

Cinnamomum Zeylanicum

Cinnamon has delighted our taste buds for centuries with its warm-sweet taste, mellow aroma and considered as one of the most valuable herb. It is believed that cinnamon was among the first used spices in the ancient era and was valued for its smell. The old version of cinnamon comes from the C. zeylanicum tree and the modern version comes from the C. cassia tree. It is said that the true form of cinnamon is native to Sri Lanka and the southeastern coast of India. The cinnamon powder actually comes from large pieces of older bark found in the lower part of the tree and this bark is stronger. The non-toxic cinnamon oil is extracted from the leaves. Cassia is known as Chinese cinnamon also and named as Cinnamomum cassia.

Cinnamon, the dried bark of the laurel tree has been used from antiquity. Though it has the distinct origin but cinnamon was widely used in ancient world. The depiction of cinnamon can be found in Chinese writing, dated back to 2800BC. In medieval periods it was used to preserve meat for its anti bacterial and anti fungal properties as well as it was also used to treat coughing, sore and hoarseness. The record says that the Egyptians used it for embalming potions, perfumes, incense and oils.

Types of Cinnamon

- Cinnamomum verum (Ceylon cinnamon- True cinnamon)
- Cinnamomum cassia (Chines cinnamon)
- Cinnamomum burmannii (Indonesian)
- Cinnamomum loureiroi (Vietamese cassia)

Chemical & medicinal properties in cinnamon bark

- Tannins - polymeric 5,7,3',4'-tetrahydroxyflavan-3,4-diol units
- Condensed Tannins - catechins and proanthocyanidins
- Procyanidins
- Resins
- Sugars
- Calcium oxalate
- Insecticidal compounds - cinnzelanin and cinnzelanol
- Coumarin
- Oil – eugenol
- Cinnzeylanine
- Catechin
- Afzelechin
- Proanthocyanidins
- Vitamin A
- Pyridoxine
- Minerals – potassium, iron, zinc, manganese and calcium

Health Benefits
Traditional medical use:

- **Ayurveda:** In ayurvedic medicine it is believed that cinnamon can be used to treat digestive disorders, to improve reproductive and respiratory system. Ayurvedic treatment displays that cinnamon can prevent cough, sinusitis and gynecologic disorders as well as pyria.
- **Traditional Chinese Medicine (TCM):** Cinnamon has been praised for having profound medicinal values in TCM. According to TCM, cinnamon has the warming effect and

thus it can increase the body temperature. In TCM, cinnamon is used to treat energy disorders, asthma and to stimulate appetite.

- **Biblical:** The medicinal value of cinnamon can be found in Bible also.
- **European:** Cinnamon bark has been used in Europe as an antispasmodic for mild gastrointestinal spasms and traditionally it has been considered as the warming herb.

Modern Medicinal Use:

- The eugenol oil property in cinnamon is considered as local anesthetic and antiseptic. Therefore it is useful to gum and dental treatment.
- It is said that cinnamon has the highest anti-oxidant strength among all food sources in nature. So, it works as anti-inflammatory or can reduce the proliferation of cancer cells. The ORAC value is 267536 TE.
- The anti-clotting properties prevent platelet clogging inside the blood vessels and prevents stroke.
- Numerous studies have stated that cinnamon regulates blood sugar in our body.
- By reducing LDL cholesterol level, cinnamon helps to reduce the risk of having cardiovascular diseases.
- The natural chemical, cinnamaldehyde in cinnamon increases progesterone and decrease testosterone in women and thus helps to maintain the balance of hormone in women.
- It is effective to reduce menstrual pain.
- The active principles in cinnamon increase the motility of the intestinal tract.
- Cinnamon prevents infections.

17. BROCCOLI SPROUTS

BRASSICA OLERACEA ITALICA

Broccoli seeds have to be moistened and left in the dark for few days to allow them for growing. So, broccoli sprouts are actually three-four days old tiny broccoli plants that contain potent nutrigenomic potential. Broccoli is the member of Cruciferous plant that also includes cabbages and cauliflower. Broccoli seeds can be stored in cool and dry place up to five years for sprouting later. The nutritional content in broccoli sprouts can vary depending on the vitamin and mineral content in the soil.

Though broccoli sprouts have found its popularity in USA after 1990's, it has thousand years old history. Raw broccoli sprouts have been embraced as a dietary staple by the health conscious people for long years. In 1992, a science team of Johns Hopkins University found glucoraphanin in broccoli. Glucoraphanin is the glucosinolate precursor of sulforaphane and is a cancer fighting phytochemical. Later, in 1997, another research has discovered that three-four day old broccoli sprouts have at least 20times more glucoraphanin concentration than full-grown broccoli.

Active Ingredients in Broccoli Sprouts

- Sulforaphane (most valuable Phytochemical)
- Top other Phytochemicals – cartenoids, lycopene, zeaxathin and lutein.
- Ascorbic acid
- Carotenoid
- Chlorophyll
- Phenol

- Minerals –Sodium, Calcium, Iron, Potassium and Magnesium
- Fiber
- Enzymes – sucrase, diastase, alpha, glycosidase and invertase.
- Vitamins – A, C and K
- Protein

Medicinal Use

Cancer-
Researchers from Johns Hopkins University School of Medicine and Bloomberg School of Public Health have observed that broccoli sprouts can help the body detoxify carcinogens. Broccoli sprouts can help to eliminate cancer-causing toxins. Sulforaphane component in broccoli sprout inhibits the growth of cancer cells and helps liver to oust the harmful toxins along with carcinogens from body. A research held in Ulster University have shown that regular eating of broccoli sprouts protects DNA from damage and lowers the risk of cancer.

- **Breast Cancer:** University of Michigan Comprehensive Cancer Center have studied that broccoli sprouts may inhibit cancerous stem cells to prevent breast cancer and shrink the existing tumor.

- **Bladder Cancer:** An extract from broccoli sprouts contains high dose of isothiocyanate in particular sulforaphane and prevents bladder cancer. Being a rich source of several isothiocyanat, broccoli sprouts lower the risk of having bladder cancer.

- **Prostrate cancer:** Regular consumption of broccoli sprouts may help to reduce the risk of prostate cancer, as it contain sulforaphane, which can prevent prostate cancer by activating some genes that can fight against cancer. "Selenium-enriched broccoli sprouts were prepared using a sodium selenite solution. Their anticancer properties were evaluated in human prostate cancer cell lines and compared with those of a control broccoli sprout extract. Selenium-enriched broccoli sprouts were superior to normal broccoli sprouts in inhibiting cell proliferation, decreasing prostate-specific antigen secretion, and inducing apoptosis of prostate cancer cells. Furthermore, selenium-enriched broccoli sprouts but, not normal broccoli sprouts, induced a downregulation of the survival Akt/mTOR pathway. Our results suggest that this enrichment could potentially be used as an alternative selenium source for prostate cancer prevention and therapy.(http://www.raysahelian.com/broccolisprouts.html).

- **Other types of cancer-** Skin cancer and Stomach Cancer.

Cardiovascular Benefits

By normalizing the blood pressure level, broccoli sprouts helps reducing cardiovascular diseases risk. A study published in "Diabetes Research and Clinical Practice" has shown that regular eating of broccoli sprouts decreases triglyceride levels and significantly a higher level of high-density lipoprotein, or HDL, the great form of cholesterol.

Arthritis

Some active compounds in broccoli sprouts may help to prevent the most common form of arthritis.

Eye Health

Active sulforaphane in broccoli sprouts may protect eyes from damage caused by chemical carcinogens and ultraviolet light.

Some Other health Benefits –

- **The useful anti-oxidant properties in broccoli sprouts help our body to detoxify the harmful enzymes.**
- **Broccoli sprouts maintain lungs health associated with COPD.**
- **Broccoli sprouts can be used to manage diabetes.**

- **It protects intestine.**
- **It prevents having Ulcer.**
- **Broccoli sprouts help to lower cholesterol levels.**
- **It can be taken to protect from** Allergy and asthma.

18. GREEN TEA

Camellia Sinensis

Green tea is made from the leaves of camellia sinensis tree. After plucking from the tree green tea leaves have to be preserved quickly and heated immediately to prevent oxidation. The minimal oxidation during processing is one of the reasons of being a healthy beverage. Both of black tea leaves and green tea leaves come from the same tree but the cultivation conditions, processing methods, fermentation and the brewing methods differentiate the characteristics and green tea, obviously, holds the distinct place for having more therapeutic properties than black tea. Though green tea originated to China and has a remarkable place in Japan but due to the flavor and health benefits, green tea has been able to find its place in different cultures throughout the world.

In 8th century, the history of green tea begun in China when the method of steaming tea leaves for preventing oxidation was introduced, At that time green tea was not meant to be for the common people, as it used to be reserved for the monks and aristocrats. During 8th-9th century AD Japanese Buddhist monks came to know about green tea along with its medical properties from the Chinese temples. Chinese people have used green tea as medicine over the centuries.

Organic Constituents of green tea

The chemical constituents or ingredients in green tea are very complex and the level of each ingredient varies depending on harvesting season, making process or changes with location. Green tea has about 200 bioactive compounds. Polyphenols are the largest compound, as well as the most important ingredient, as they contain ant-oxidant properties (flavonoids). Chinese and Japanese green tea do not contain higher level of polyphenols. That is why Chinese and Japanese green tea taste good, as higher level of polyphenols make a bad green tea but it does not make it less healthier.

- **Polyphenols- these are the most important green tea nutrients.**
- **Catachins** (important polyphenol)
  Epicatechin
  Epicatechin-3-gallate
  Epigallocatechin
  And
  EGCG(Epigallocatechin-3-gallate)**:** The higher concentration of EGCG can be found in green tea and it is the most active ingredient.

- Flavonoids- flavonols are found maximum
- Other polyphenols.
- Caffeine.
- Theanines.
- **Theophylline.**
- **Theobromine**
- **Fat.**
- **Wax.**
- **Saponins.**
- **Essential oils.**
- **Carotine.**
- Vitamins – A, B1, B12, C, K and P.
- Minerals – Fluoride, Iron, Calcium, Copper, Nickel, Zinc, Magnesium, Strontium, Manganese and Aluminum.
- **Molybdenum**
- **Phosphorus**

Polyphenols factor in Green tea

Green tea is the bag full of polyphenols and the EGCG catechin polyphenol plays the key role to our health, as EGCG is a powerful anti-oxidant. Fortunately, the higher concentration of EGCG can be found in green tea and it is the most active ingredient also. It has been proved that EGCG is 100 times more effective in neutralizing free radicals than vitamin C and 25 times more powerful than vitamin E.

This catechin inhibits the growth of cancer, as well as it can kill the cancer cells without harming the living cells. EGCG can also helpful to lower the LDL cholesterol level. Researchers from the University of Kansas have stated that EGCG is more powerful than resveratrol.

Why we should drink green tea regularly!

· **It maintains our oral health:**

Active polyphenols along with the natural fluoride in green tea kill the bacteria that cause of tooth decay, gum disease, bad breath and tooth loss. Without any added sweetener, green tea serves this purpose to the fullest.

· **It prevents cancer:**

The active EGCG and other anti-oxidant agents can protect us from cancer. The density of cancer is low in Japan, as they take green tea regularly. Not only it prevents cancer but also fights against the growth of cancer cells by inhibiting it and kills the cancer cells.

Green tea is helpful to prevent- breast cancer, bladder cancer, lung cancer, ovarian cancer, esophageal cancer, colorectal cancer, prostate cancer, pancreatic cancer, stomach cancer and skin cancer.

· **Green tea improves bone health as well as keeps arthritis away:**

The fluoride and calcium content keep our bones strong. Green tea can help prevent and reduce the risk of rheumatoid arthritis. Green tea has benefit for your health as it protects the cartilage by blocking the enzyme that destroys cartilage.

- **It prevents Atherosclerosis:**
  The anti oxidant properties in green tea may protect us from having Atherosclerosis.

- Green tea significantly reduces blood levels of harmful LDL cholesterol.
- It is very helpful to treat Diabetes.
- Population-based clinical studies have shown that men who drink more than 10 cups of green tea per day are less likely to develop liver problems.
- It can be the cause of Weight Loss.
- Drinking green tea is helpful to maintain good cardiovascular health and it lowers the risk of heart attack.

- Green tea helps boost your memory. And although there's no cure for Alzheimer's it helps slow the process of reduced acetylcholine in the brain, which leads to Alzheimer's.
- The anti-oxidant properties protect our skin from the harmful effect of free radicals.
- It can be used as anti-aging medicine.
- People drinking green tea also are less likely to progress with Parkinson's.
- It strengthens our immunity system.
- Green tea is very much helpful for lowering the high blood pressure.
- **Other disease that can be treated or prevented by drinking green tea:** Flu, Asthma, Allergies, Stress, Herpes and ear infection etc.

19. HIMALAYAN SEA SALT

Rock Salt

Himalayan salt is considered as the most pure form of salt available on the earth. This salt is derived from the ancient sea salt deposits in Himalayas. It has never been exposed to the outer impurities, as it has been protected deep inside the Himalayas for millions of year. Himalayan Salt was formed from the primordial ocean during a time of great tectonic pressure. This crystal salt is absolutely pristine and natural, identical in composition to the ancient primal ocean. Deepening on the ingredients, this salt varies in color from sheer shade of white deep reds and various shades of pink.

This extraordinary salt has been treated as a valuable commodity for centuries and the Himalayan people have used it as preservative. This salt is still extracted using the traditional system. From the extracting to the packaging all is done by hand without seeking help from any of modern mechanisms. Khewra salt mines situated in Pakistan supply the maximum of this salt to the world markets.

Himalayan salt contains most of the minerals that are necessary for our health; it includes macro minerals and trace minerals. Himalayan salt contains some minerals that are toxic in large quantities, including lead and plutonium, but which are safe in trace amounts 100% pure Himalayan salt contains 84 natural elements and those are –

1) Hydrogen, 2) Lithium, 3) Beryllium, 4) Boron, 5) Carbon, 6) Nitrogen, 7) Oxygen, 8) Fluoride, 9) Sodium, 10) Magnesium, 11) Aluminum, 12) Silicon, 13) Phosphorus, 14) Sulfur, 15) Chloride, 16) Calcium, 17) Scandium, 18) Titanium, 19) Vanadium, 20) Chromium, 21) Manganese, 22) Iron, 23) Cobalt, 24) Nickel, 25) Copper, 26) Zinc, 27) Gallium, 28) Germanium, 29) Arsenic, 30) Selenium, 31) Bromine, 32) Rubidium, 33) Strontium, 34) Yttrium, 35) Zirconium, 36) Niobium, 37) Molybdenum, 38) Ruthenium, 39) Rhodium 40) Palladium, 41) Silver, 42) Cadmium, 43) Indium, 44) Tin, 45) Antimony, 46)

Tellurium, 47) Iodine, 48) Cesium, 49) Barium, 50) Lanthanum, 51) Cerium, 52) Praseodymium, 53) Samarium, 54) Europium, 55) Gadolinium, 56) Terbium, 57) Dysprosium, 58) Holmium, 59) Erbium, 60) Thulium, 61) Ytterbium, 62) Lutetium, 63) Hafnium, 64) Tantalum, 65) Tungsten, 66) Rhenium, 67) Osmium, 68) Iridium, 69) Platinum, 70) Gold, 71) Mercury, 72) Thallium, 73) Lead, 74) Bismuth, 75) Polonium, 76) Astatine, 77) Francium, 78) Radium, 79) Actinium, 80) Thorium, 81) Protactinium, 82) Uranium, 83) Neptunium and 84) Plutonium.

Medicinal Use

Regular consumption of Himalayan salt provides essential minerals and trace elements that your body requires. It also balances electrolytes, assists in balancing the body's pH and increases circulation and conductivity. Even, consuming a gram of Himalayan salt per day can help our body's metabolic process and help to reduce any deposits that have built up in the arteries. Himalayan crystal salt can be used directly to the foods or can be taken as brine.

Himalayan salt is considered healthier than regular table salt, which often has additives, such as the anti-caking agent Sodium Ferro cyanide.

- It promotes bone strength.
- Regular use of few drops of brine can support libido.
- It assists in the cellular absorption of minerals.
- It helps to improve the connective tissue in the organs.
- It helps to regulate the water content throughout our body.
- Himalayan salt promotes a healthy pH balance in your cells, particularly our brain cells.
- It also prevents muscle cramps.
- It brings about significant improvements in the respiratory, circulatory, and nervous systems.
- It helps the procedure of absorption of food particles through intestinal tract.
- This crystal salt promotes blood sugar health and can be used as anti-aging agent.
- Surprisingly it promotes sleep naturally.

- It is also contains some essential properties to maintain cardiovascular health and to prevent arthritis.
- The most important benefit is that it helps to fulfill the requirement of some essential minerals.

20. SOUR SOP

Annona muricata

Sour sop fruit belongs to the *Annonaceae family and comes from Annona genus. It is native to Caribbean islands, along with South America and grows naturally on tropical areas in Asia also. Though sour sop is famous worldwide, the fresh version can be hardly found outside of tropical areas. If the careful protection from frost during winter can be given, sour sop can survive in the continental United States also.*

The indigenous people of the Amazon Basin used to take all parts of sour sop tree, including, leaves, bark, root, fruit and seeds as remedy for various ailments. They believed that regular consumption of sour sip tea might increase the quality of life. It is said that it was one of the first fruit trees carried from America to the Old World Tropics where it has become widely distributed from southeastern China to Australia and the warm lowlands of eastern and western Africa.

Common Names: Coração de Boi, Aluguntugui, Guanábana, Adunu, Brazilian pawpaw, Nangka londa and nangka blanda.

Chemical and Nutritional Properties

· Fruit

Glucose, Fructose, Vitamins(C, B1, B2), Magnesium, Iron, Sodium, Fósforo, Asimilobine, Anoniine, Potasio, Fiber, Protein and Arginine.

· Leaf

Lactonas- Annohexocina; Annomuricina A, B, C y E; Annomutacina; Annopentocinas A, B and C; Muricoreacina; Gigantetronemina; Murihexocina A and C; Javoricina.

Isoquinolinas- Anonaine, Anoniine, Atherospermine, Coreximine

Lipidos- Stearic acid, Gentisic acid, Lignoceric acid and Linoleic acid.

· Seeds

Lactonas, Annomonicina, Annomontacina, Annonacina, Annomuricatina, Annonacinona and Javoricina

On sheet of *Annona muricata* is a group of substances called **acetogenins to which they attribute most of the health benefits of soursop, including the anti-cancer effect.
- Bullatacin
- Bullatacinone
- Muricoreacin
- Murihexocin C
- A Annomuricin
- Annomuricin B
- A Muricatocin
- Muricatocin C
- Muricapentocin

Health Benefits

The fruits and leaves can be used as the remedy for various diseases, including, fever, distress, and respiratory problems etc. According to Memorial Sloan-Kettering Cancer Center, sour sop contains number of natural substances, which have biological activities. A study published in Journal of Ethno pharmacology have depicted that an extract of sour sop inhibited the growth of Herpes virus in the laboratory.

Cancer: In laboratory research it has been found that sour sop extract can kill certain types of breast and liver cancer cells that are resistant to chemotherapy drugs. The medicinal properties in sour sop can effectively target and kill malignant cells in 12 types of cancer, including, colon, breast, prostate, lung and pancreatic cancer.

Kills Parasites: In an assessment of Graviola, published in the December 2008 issue of the "Journal of Dietary Supplements" by U.S. researchers Lana Dvorkin-Camiel and Julia S. Whelan, multiple in-vitro studies determined that Graviola is effective against various microbial and parasitic agents.

Helps to strengthen immune system: Acetogenins, annocatacin, annocatalin, annohexocin, annonacin, annomuricin, anomurine, anonol, caclourine, gentisic acid, gigantetronin, linoleic acid and muricapentocin are found in sour sop. These are those substances, which can improve our immune system

It is source of High vitamin C: Regular eating habit of sour sop fruit fulfill the requirement of vitamin C in our body. The content of vitamin C is high enough on sour sop is an excellent antioxidant to increase endurance and slow the aging process.

Other healthe Benefits:

*Along with soursop fruit, the bark, leaves and roots of the soursop trees are popularly used as ingredients in various traditional herbal medicines. Soursop leaves health benefits include calming the nerves. Tea prepared with soursop leaves works as a pain reliever. The sap of its leaves, or the flesh, can be applied topically to get rid of eczema, skin rash and swelling. Topical application promotes fast healing of wounds and prevents infections.

* The leaf decoction is effective for head lice and bedbugs.
* The juice when taken when fasting, it is believed to relieve liver ailments and leprosy.
* It can prevent osteoporosis.
* Regular consumption may help to avoid nerve damage and can maintain heart health.
* It also prevents bacterial infections.
* The root bark can be used as an antidote for poisoning.

21. RED WINE

History says that the earlier productions of red wine were taken place during 600BC in the Caucasus region between Europe and Asia. The people from Egypt and Rome used to ferment grape juice and preserved for up to 25 years in order to have better quality res wine. At the very beginning of second 11th century AD the culture of red win was brought to England from the Bordeaux region. Later this red wine came to United States with the European immigrants. Ohio and New York were the first states to produce red wine in US.

Types of red wine:
1) Merlot – It was invented in first century in France.
2) Pinot Nior- It was from ancient Rome.
3) Chianti- this Italian red wine was invented before 15th century.
4) Sangiovese- Arround 1722AD it was invented in Tuscany.
5) Zinfandel- This is the youngest counterpart among all the types of wine and invented in USA during mid 19th century.

There are also various types of wine available around the world, such as Malbec and Syrah.

Constituents in Red Wine:

- Carbohydrates.
- Fructose.
- Glucose.
- Acids- Malic, Tartaric, Lactic and Acetic.
- Pectins.
- Ethanol.
- Alchohol.
- Phenolics.
- Glycerol.
- Tannins.

- Anthocyanins.
- Inorganic constituents.
- Nitrogenous compounds.
- Potassium.
- Anions.
- Cations.

Red Wine and Resveratol- Health benefits

Resveratol is a natural occurring polyphenos, which has powerful anti-oxidant properties and can be found in red wine. On the Resveratol part we have discussed about the health benefits of resveratol. As a huge source of resveratol, red wine derives all the health benefits from it.

- Due to the anti-oxidant resveratol, consuming a moderate amount of red wine daily can maintain the good heart health and prevent the artery from damages. The huge amount of reveratol in red wine increases the HDL cholesterol level. Flavonoids in red wine also protect us from having cardiovascular disease.
- Moderate amount of regular red wine consumption can protect from cancer. Along with the resveratol and other anti-oxidant properties, red wine can inhibit the growth of cancer cells.
- Red wine prevents tooth decay. The polyphenols components in red wine protect gums from diseases.
- The anti-oxidant properties prevent the oxidative damage, which can be the cause of Alzheimer's and type-2 diabetes.
- The resveratol in red wine elevates some specific enzyme levels and protect our brain during stroke.
- Red wine helps to reduce blood clotting in vessels.

22. MUSHROOM

Agaricus bisporus

According to hieroglyphics of 4600 years ago, ancient Egyptian people used to praise mushrooms as the plant of immortality. The pharaohs in Egypt did not allow common people to consume mushrooms as it were reserved for the royal use only. The culture of mushrooms was practiced worldwide for over centuries including, Russia, China, Greece, Mexico and Latin America. In the early civilizations France was the leader in formal cultivation of mushrooms. The English people borrowed the practice of culturing mushrooms from France. In 19th century mushroom has made its way to the United Sates. After much experimentation USA mushrooms industries have begun to grow. In 1924, the Pennsylvania Department of Agriculture boasted that 85% of U.S. mushrooms were grown in Pennsylvania.

Mushrooms are actually fungi but all the fungi should not be considered as mushrooms. Mushrooms are of the fungi family subdivision of Basidiomycotina, of the class Hymenomycetes. Mushrooms are actually the fruits of the fungal body and contain mushroom "seeds" called spores. The rest of the fungal organism typically lives in the soil, wood, or some other material and is composed of thread-like strands known as mycelium. In nature some myceliums may spreads over hundreds of square miles. Many mushroom-producing species are important decomposers, particularly of wood. These species are often relatively easy to cultivate. However, many species have a special, symbiotic, "mycorrhizal" relationship with particular species of plants. Often, neither the mushroom nor the plant will grow without a mycorrhizal partner.

Mushrooms have their own kingdom apart from that of plants and animals. Mushrooms obtain their nutrition by metabolizing non-living organic things, as they do not have chlorophyll and most of them are considered saprophytes. The body stores the nutrients along with other essential elements and under the comfortable condition it begin to fruit.

Mushrooms have not only been enriching the recipes of culinary arts but also they have found their distinctive place for their medicinal values. More than twenty species of mushrooms are cultivated commercially to fulfill the supply for pharmaceutical industries and food demands. All the wild mushrooms are not edible, as it may be the cause of toxic effect.

Here are some types of edible Mushrooms & Their Health Benefits

1) Turkey Tail Mushroom (Trametes versicolor)

Turkey tail mushrooms are one of the most researched and respected of the medicinal mushroom. This type of mushrooms is very common in United States. Turkey tail is common bracket fungi and has no stalk like other mushrooms. Turkey tail mushrooms have the long history of medicinal use in China and Japan; there it is called Yun and Kawaratake, respectively.

Constituents: β-glucan-proteins (Coriolan, PSK), Polysaccharide K (PSK), Ergosterol (provitamin D2), Polysaccharopeptide (PSP).

Health benefits-
· The Polysaccharopeptide (PSP) in turkey tail is effective in targeting prostate cancer stem cells and suppressing tumor formation.
· It is a powerful anti-oxidant.
· It helps strengthening the immune system.

- The turkey tail mushroom has the immense power to fight against cancer and protects the uninfected cells.
- Turkey tail may also improve quality of life by reducing susceptibility to infections and other negative effects of having a suppressed immune system.
- It helps to remove chronic congestion.

2) Maitake Mushrooms (Grifola frondosa)

This mushroom is also called as hen of the woods and native to Japan and North America. This polypore mushroom is often found growing in clumps around the base of oak trees; maitake mushroom can reach a weight of 50 pounds. Like the sulphur shelf mushroom, G. frondosa is a perennial fungus that often grows in the same place for a number of years in succession. For thousands of years the Asian people have used maitake mushrooms in tonics, soups, teas, prepared foods, and herbal formulas to promote health and long life.

Health benefits-
- **Cacner:**Dr. Shari Lieberman, the author of the book "Maitake Mushroom and D-Fraction" have stated that Maitake D-fraction may inhibit cancer development and spread and also make chemotherapy drugs more effective. Maitake mushrooms contain the beta-glucan polysaccharide (grifolan), for which these mushrooms has the ability to block the growth of cancer tumors and it help to stimulate the immune systems of breast cancer patients.
- **Anti-diabetic:** Early animal studies suggest that maitake mushroom extract may lower blood sugar levels and improve insulin sensitivity, as well as increase levels of insulin in the blood.
- According to University of Wisconsin Botany Department maitake mushrooms modulates the cytokines, produced by the white blood corpuscle to boost the immune response.
- Maitake mushrooms help to prevent *Ovulation disorders*.
- It helps to lower the cholesterol level in blood.
- It also has the properties to fight against HIV.

- Maitake can be the best chemotherapy support.
- It protects us from chronic fatigue syndrome (CFS).

3) Shiitake Mushrooms (Lentinula edodes)

Common names: Lentinula edodes, Oriental Black mushrooms, Forest mushrooms, Chinese mushrooms and Golden oak mushroom.

Shiitake mushrooms have been used medicinally in China for about more than 6000 years. According to Traditional Chinese theory, Chinese people praise it more like animal rather than a plant and even it has a social aspect in their lives also. This mushroom is equally famous in America for its slightly spongy texture, with a rich 'meaty' flavor and exotic taste, though these mushrooms do not grow wild in USA but have been cultivated commercially over past few decades.

Constituents: lentinan, eritadenine, iron, vitamin C, protein, Lenthionine L-ergothioneine, thiamine, riboflavin, niacin, B2, B12, and high levels of vitamin D.

Health benefits-

- **Cancer:** The lentinan constituent in shiitake mushroom helps to prevent cancer as well as inhibits the infected cancer cells. Researchers have speculated that more than 100 different types of compounds in shiitake mushrooms may work together to accomplish these anti-tumor results.
- **Immunity booster:** This is the most effective benefit found in laboratory research. The effective compound lentinan can strengthen our immune system other than fighting against cancer. It is believed that shiitake mushrooms are more effective than any prescribed drug fighting against influenza and other ailments.

- **Thrombosis preventive:** The high level of lenthionine in shiitake mushroom prevents thrombosis in veins and maintains the health of vein.
- It maintains the cardiovascular health.
- The eritadenine compound in shiitake mushroom is thought to lower cholesterol by blocking the way cholesterol is absorbed into the bloodstream
- It can be an aid to weight loss.
- Plenty of shiitake mushrooms in regular diet help to increase the level of iron in blood.

4) Chaga Mushrooms (Inonotus obliquus)

In Siberia it is addressed as "Gift from God" while Chinese people praise it as "King of Plants" and known as "Diamond of the Forest" in Japan.

Chaga mushrooms are unique and different from other types of mushrooms. It is hard like a wood, rather than soft as other mushrooms. It has the appearance of a black, irregular, cracked mass, grows on tree trunks. Chaga is actually a parasitic mushroom that grows mainly in birch trees. Chaga is the most nutritionally dense of all tree growths. To survive in harsh climates, chaga concentrates natural compounds for its protection, and that is why it is so powerful. It is experienced that among all the chaga mushrooms, he Siberian counterpart contains more superior grade medicinal properties.

Active ingredients:
- **Phytochemicals-** Chaga mushroom contains over 215 phytochemicals, which are thought to be the anti-oxidants and promote human health.
- Polysaccharides.
- Beta Glucan.
- Betulin or Betulinic Acid.
- Betulinic Acid

- Polysaccharides
- Tripeptides
- Inotodiol
- Triterpenes
- Sterols
- Saponins
- Trametenolic Acid
- Lanosterols.
- Flavonoids
- Melanin
- Amino Acids
- Minerals- Calcium, Copper, Iron, Manganese, Magnesium, Zinc, Phosphorus and Potassium.
- Vitamins- B1, B2, B3, B5, C, D2 and K.

Health Benefits

Chaga are a nutrient dense fungus, containing flavonoids, sterols, polysaccharides, polyphenols, essential minerals, and vitamins. Another compound present in Chaga, beta glucan, is believed to activate T-cell activity, and increase production of antibodies. South Korean researchers from Kyunghee University evaluated the efficacy of chaga in preventing damage to DNA. Cells were treated with an extract made from chaga mushrooms and then exposed to oxidative stress. Of the cells treated with chaga, there was 40 percent less damage to DNA structure, in comparison to the untreated cells. (http://healing.answers.com/herbs/the-health-benefits-of-chaga-mushrooms).

- In Traditional Chinese Medicine chaga is regarded as the longevity factor.
- **Cancer:** Chaga contains betulinic acid, which is a powerful cytotoxic and triggers apoptosis through a direct effect on the mitochondria of cancer cells. Chaga can help to prevent cancer.
- It is a powerful anti-oxidant.
- Chaga works as anti HIV agent.

- It improves immune system.
- Chaga promote cellular respiration and proliferation.
- Some active properties in chaga prevent candida.
- Chaga is an adaptogen, which means its compounds increase the body's ability to adapt to stress, fatigue, anxiety and changing situations.
- **Other diseases that can be treated or prevented by chaga:** Diabetes, Crohn's Disease, Hepatoprotective, Heart Disease, Gastric, Hodgkin's Lymphoma, Pulmonary Diseases, Skin and Stomach ailments, Tuberculosis, Ulcerative Colitis (UC), Arthritis, Asthma and Influenza.

5) Reishi Mushrooms (Ganoderma lucidum)

Reishi mushrooms are hard as wood and have bitter taste; that is why these are not often used in cooking. Reishi mushrooms are mainly cultivated for medicinal purpose. Reishi mushroom has been used as valuable natural herb in eastern Asia for thousands of years.

Ingredients: Reishi mushrooms contain a group of triterpenes along with a wide spectrum of beneficial polysaccharides. Apart from those, various alkaloids are also found in reishi extract.

Health Benefits:
- It is believed that reishi mushrooms are non toxic and can be taken regularly without having any side effect.
- Several studies have shown that reishi mushrooms have anti-carcinogenic, anti-tumor, and immunotherapeutic effects.
- Studies indicated that ganoderic acids help alleviate common allergies by inhibiting histamine release, improve oxygen utilization and improve liver functions.
- **Some diseases that can be treated or prevented by consuming reishi mushrooms-** Asthma, Bronchitis, Aids,

Prostate cancer, cardiovascular disease, Fatigue, Ulcers, Viral infections, High blood pressure and kidney disorders etc.

6) Agaricus Blazei (Agaricus subrufescens)

Agaricus Blazei is native to Brazil and knows as *"Cogumelo do Sol"* there. Over the years this mushroom is considers as one of the most important edible and culinary-medicinal biotechnological species. This mushroom grows with a cap, whose color varies from reddish, grey to brown.

Health Benefits:
· Complex polysaccharides isolated from Agaricus blazei like beta-glucans have been found in laboratory studies to inhibit tumor growth and directly kill cancer cells. Other studies also suggest the ability of Agaricus blazei extract to inhibit cancer metastases.
· Further research confirms the ability of the Agaricus Blazei mushroom to lower blood cholesterol, inhibit the negative effects of pathogens and also deter angiogenesis. Other animal and clinical research indicates that the mushroom can lower blood sugar and control insulin.
· Beta-glucans in Blazei mushroom helps boosting the body immunity system.
· It has anti-oxidant properties, which can prevent free radicals.
· It is an aid to diabetes patients.
· It helps to improve circulatory problems and digestive problems.
· Agaricus Blazei can be used as anti carcinogen.

7) Lions Mane Mushrooms (Hericium erinaceus)

These globular-shaped mushrooms sport cascading teeth-like spines rather than the more common gills and white in color. In place of the traditional mushroom cap is a large clump of teeth, which are spine-like structures a few millimeters long. These teeth actually manufacture and release the spores. These mushrooms provide a vast array of potential medicinal compounds and have been used in Traditional Chinese Medicine. The tea made from Lion's Mane mushrooms has been used for centuries in traditional Japanese herbals, primarily as a "tonic".

Active ingredients:
· Polysaccharides
· Fatty acids
· Polypeptides
· Oleanolic acids
· Adenosine

Health benefits:

· Improves the brain functions.
· Protects against cancer.
· Improves immunity power.
· Has an anti-inflammatory effect.
· It has the positive effects on dementia.
· Prevents from breakdown of healthy neurological function.

8) Meshima Mushrooms (Phellinus linteus)

Mesima mushroom is found on wild mulberry trees. Mesima contains protein bounded polysaccharides. It enhances immunological activities. Mesima is being studies for anti-cancer activities.

Uniquely among the medicinal mushrooms, the Chinese Pharmacopoeia describes the energy of P. linteus as Cold (see section on Medicinal Mushrooms According to Traditional Chinese

Medicine) and ascribes to it an extensive range of indications, including: cancer, diabetes, HIV, angina,leucorrhoea, diarrhoea and accelerated wound healing.

- Acidic polysaccharide from Phellinus linteus inhibits melanoma cell metastasis by blocking cell adhesion and invasion.
- The acidic polysaccharide (PL) from Phellinus linteus is an immunostimulator that has therapeutic activity against cancers.
- It has anti-inflammatory actions.
- It can prevent Rheumatoid Arthritis
- **Korean researchers showed that Phellinus linteus significantly inhibited melanoma cell metastasis in mice. In the study, Phellinus linteus directly inhibited cancer cell adhesion to and invasion through the extracellular matrix.**

9) Cordyceps Mushrooms (Cordiceps sinensis)

According to Chinese history this natural herb was reserved for the emperors only, as it was very much rare. The Traditional Chinese Medicine has used it to treat cough, impotence, fatigue and cancer. This mushroom is known as "winter worm, summer grass" and "Chinese caterpillar mushroom". It grows generally in high altitude levels and in cold, grassy, alpine meadows of the Himalayan Mountains.

Cordyceps militaris constitutes the highest amount of nutritional components among the 400 species in the genus *Cordyceps*. It is actually produced from a parasitic relationship between fungus and larva, usually that of a moth. After infecting the larva, the fungus forms the mycelium which mummifies the body while consuming the larva.

Active Ingredients:
- Kordisftit acid (D-mannitol)
- Gamma amino butyric acid (GABA)
- Polysaccharides
- Stanins
- Enzymes

Health benefits:
- It has been seen that Cordyceps mushrooms have the enormous energy boosting ability, as well as it promotes longevity.
- It is studied that consuming of cordyceps mushrooms improve the quality of life and immune system after cancer chemotherapy.
- **The diseases that can be treated or prevented by cordyceps mushrooms:** sexual dysfunctions, Fatigue, Anemia, Liver disorders, Bronchitis, Kidney disorders, High cholesterol and Heart arrhythmias.

10) Enokitake Mushrooms (Flammulina velutipes)

Enokitake mushrooms or Enoki Mushrooms are very popular in Asian cuisine, especially in Japan for its nice crunchy feels and delicious flavors. It grows naturally on stumps of *Enoki* or the Chinese Hackberry tree and on the wood of quaking aspen and other poplars (members of the genus Populus) in western North America. These long stemmed mushrooms with white tiny caps resemble bean sprouts. On the contrary wild enoki mushrooms have black stems and broad brown caps.

Common Name:
Wild Enokitake Mushrooms -Winter Mushrooms, Velvet Stems, Velvet Mushrooms and Velvet Foot.

Cultivated Enokitake Mushrooms -Lily Mushrooms and Golden Needle Mushrooms.

Health Benefits:

- It has been cited that who takes Enokitake mushrooms regularly, has significantly lower risk of cancer.
- These mushrooms contain anti-oxidant (ergothioneine) properties and that is why these mushrooms are helpful to fight against cancer, free radicals and boost immune system. Other tumor fighting compounds also give it other medicinal values.
- Enoki mushrooms are the great source of minerals, protein, vitamins and dietary fiber.
- The beta-glucans (long-chain polysaccharides) in enoki mushrooms are beneficial to human immune system and can prevent diabetes, asthma and allergies.
- It is anti viral and anti bacterial.
- Enokitake can fight against Alzheimer's and dementia.
- Regular consumption of these mushrooms can prevent gastro enteric ulcers and liver disease.

11)Artist's Conk mushrooms (Ganoderma applanatum)

Artist's conk is exceptionally common in Maine growing on older sugar maples and many other hardwood trees usually persisting for years. When they are picked the interior reveals layers of pores that are like rings on a tree in describing age. Artist's Conk gets its name from the change in color which occurs when the white underside of the conk is scratched. The scratched trace immediately turns brown, allowing artists to create intricate drawings on this natural "canvas." It is also known as a "shelf fungus" because the fruiting body forms a stalkless shelf on the sides of trees and logs. These are polypore fungi and most of them are not edible for their woody, rubbery or fibrous textures.

These mushrooms are not only native to the North East but these are in majority of the Canadian and American forests also.

Health Benefits:

- Many modern science researches have shown that the extracts from Artist's conk mushrooms can fight against cancers.
- These mushrooms can lower the level of glucose in blood and thus it is an excellent remedy for the patients suffering from diabetes.
- It also can help full to lower the blood lipid.
- The polysaccharide properties prevent the gastric ulcer.
- These mushrooms are anti-bacterial, anti-viral, anti-parasitic, immune enhancing, diuretic, and potently antioxidant.

23. PROBIOTICS

Probiotics are live microorganisms such as bacteria or yeast that are similar to beneficial microorganisms found in the human gut and they are called "friendly bacteria" or good bacteria". These microorganisms may help with digestion and offer protection from harmful bacteria, just as the existing "good" bacteria in our body do. We need these probiotics inside our body for their various beneficial actions and human digestive system contains more than 400 different species of microorganisms.

In the very beginning of 20th century the Russian Scientist Metchnikoff (Nobel Prize Owner) first discovered the presence of probiotics. He observed the long life of Bulgarian peasants, who consumed fermented milk foods and he suggested that lactobacilli might counteract the putrefactive effects of gastrointestinal metabolism. After Metchnikoff's death in 1916, the centre of activity moved to the United States. It was reasoned that bacteria originating from the gut were more likely to produce the desired effect in the gut, and in 1935 certain strains of *"Lactobacillus acidophilus"* were found to be very active when implanted in the human digestive tract.

The presences of probiotics in human guts help to regulate the immune system. These friendly bacteria sometimes get altered or destroyed by antibiotics or poor life style and the degradations of these friendly bacteria may be the cause of poor health or different ailments. Treatment with probiotics has a whole range of biochemical effects and that these effects differ markedly between the two probiotics strains, Lactobacillus paracasei and Lactobacillus rhamnosus. Adding 'friendly' bacteria can change the makeup of the bugs in the gut, not only because this increases the number of such bacteria, but also because the 'friendly' bacteria works with other bacteria in the gut, amplifying their effects. Probiotics can improve intestinal function and maintain the integrity of the lining of the intestines.

- *Lactobacillus bulgaricus* helps to convert lactose and other sugars into lactic acid, which may be particularly helpful for those who are lactose intolerant.
- *Lactobacillus acidophilus* and *Lactobacillus casei* convert lactose into lactic acid and help lactose intolerant.
- *L. Acidophilus* may also be helpful at reducing cholesterol levels.
- *Bifidobacteria is called family bacteria and it can prevent, as well as can treat various* gastrointestinal disorders, irritable bowel syndrome and constipation.

We should take probiotics supplements or probiotics foods not only for amplifying the effects of the already present probiotics in our guts but also for treating or preventing some disease. Some factors, both intrinsic and extrinsic, may influence the survival of probiotics in food –

- Dryness in a food product keeps the bacteria in a relatively quiescent state during storage, while a wet product establishes potentially active metabolism. So, the physiological state is the important factor the survival of the probiotics.
- The lower the temperature the more stable probiotics viability in the food product will be.
- Maximum probiotics cannot survive in low pH level but some bacteria like Lactobacilli and bifidobacteria can tolerate lower pH levels because they produce organic acid and products from carbohydrate metabolism.
- The higher moisture levels and water activity, the lower survival of probiotics. There is a substantial interaction between water activity and temperature with respect to their impact on the survival of quiescent probiotics.
- Obviously, the inclusion of antimicrobial preservatives can inhibit probiotics survival and elevated levels of ingredients such as salt, organic acids, and nitrates can inhibit probiotics

during storage, while starter cultures can sometimes inhibit the growth of probiotics during fermentation through the production of specific bacteriocins.

- The damages made to cell membranes by freezing probiotics are detrimental to survival, and also can make the cells more vulnerable to environmental stresses.
- The growth of bifidobacteria can be improved by the presence of suitable companion cultures, which can aid in protein hydrolysis and through the production of growth factors.

24. KEFIR

The word Kefir is derived from the Turkish word "Keif" describing a state of feeling good. Kefir is made by fermenting dairy milk through a specific mixture of yeast culture. For the fermentation process, kefir grains, a special kind of grains, are used and they look like small, lumpy granules, similar in appearance to cauliflower. According to Real Food Fermentation by Alex Lewin, Kefir grains are combinations of yeasts and bacteria living on a substrate made up of a variety of dairy components.

Though yogurt and kefir tastes like same but they differ from each other and they differ based on the type of cultures used to ferment the milk. Yogurt uses only bacteria, primarily lactobacillus species, while kefir uses both bacteria and yeast. Although yogurt can range in texture from a thick liquid to a semi solid, gel-like consistency, kefir is primarily liquid.

The grains of Kefir were considered a gift from God among the common folk and it is said that the grains were blessed by the prophet Mohammed himself. Kefir is the oldest known fermented milk drink, which originated in the Caucasus Mountains, more than 2000 years ago. The history of Kefir, outside the Caucasus Mountains is hardly known and very foggy, although we can find a little description of kefir in Marco Polo's travel accounts. In the late 19th century, the first scientific studies on Kefir were published. Though, this delicious healthy drink is recently gaining its popularity in United States, it has already found its popular place over the years in Russia, South East Asia and Northern Europe.

Health benefits:

- Kefir is considered as the strongest side-effects free natural antibiotic and strongest natural remedy for allergy.
- Kefir is a rich source of vitamins, such as A, B2, B12, D and K.
- Kefir contains essential amino acids and tryptophan, which are beneficial to our health.

- The enzymes in kefir help improving the digestive system.
- The pregnant women should drink kefir regularly, as it can inhibit the overgrowth of Group B Beta Strep bacteria.
- Because of the antibiotic and antifungal properties, kefir can treat various ailments.
- Kefir can improve immune system.
- It is very helpful to inhibit the growth of cancer cells.
- It lowers the LDL cholesterol level and cleans the gastrointestinal tract.
- Kefir alleviates intestinal disorders and promotes bowel movement.
- Kefir can protect from having prostate cancer.
- The healthy microorganisms help to maintain the proper digestive function.
- Diseased that can be treated or prevented by kefir – kidney stones, acne, parodontosis, heart disease, lung infections, chronic intestine infections, liver infections, sclerosis, anemia, asthma, bronchitis.
- Kefir normalizes metabolism and very helpful to weight loss.

25. TURMERIC ROOT

In traditional Ayurveda medicine, turmeric root has been considered as one of the most valuable herb from thousands of years. The ancient Hawaiian people used it to treat sinus infection and gastrointestinal ulcer. Turmeric was first cultivated to use as a dye and later the herbal benefits have been found. In Marco Polo's travel account it was stated turmeric root as Indian saffron served the purpose dying cloths. The medicinal properties were being disregarded by the western world until researchers from Germany have discovered the therapeutic use of turmeric root in mid 20th century. In Traditional Chinese Medicine it was valuable for its anti-inflammatory properties. Other than the herbal use, turmeric root has been used in many cuisines as food coloring and to protect foods from infections. The turmeric powder is actually made by grinding the dried turmeric roots.

Health Benefits

- **Cancer:** Curcumin is the powerful ingredient, which gives turmeric root the anti-oxidant value. It helps to protect from free radicals. This curcumin contains the potent levels of phytochemicals, polyphenols and anti-carcinogenics. Researchers at the University of Texas MD Anderson Cancer Center have studied that curcumin can inhibit the growth of cancer cells. It has also been found that this property is very potent to reduce breast cancer. Curcumin activates the human glutathione, which can inhibit cellular mutagens and prohibit the promotion of cancer cells.

  "Curcumin has been found to influence over 60 molecular targets in the cancer process. With an established safety record and a fraction of the cost of conventional chemotherapy, plant compounds like curcumin represent an enormous and almost untapped resource for cancer treatment." — Jonathan Treasure, co-founder of Centre for Natural Healing, co-author of Herb, Nutrient, and Drug Interactions: Clinical Implications and Therapeutic Strategies.

The raw turmeric root or powder is the best for serving the quality medicinal purposes.

- Curcumin also very useful to treat dyspepsia.
- Turmeric root is considered as one of the most potent natural anti-inflammatory.
- It detoxifies liver.
- Turmeric root is a natural antiseptic and natural antibacterial.
- It helps to remove amyloyd plaque buildup in the brain and thus it prevents from Alzheimer's.
- Scientists have discovered that turmeric root has the ability to inhibit cox-2 and it works as natural pain killer.
- Turmeric looks after heart health reducing cholesterol level.
- It is useful to stop internal and external bleeding.
- Turmeric roots can fight against hepatitis virus.
- Turmeric helps to re-build the skin and speeds up the wound healing.

26. KALE

Kale has been consumed for over 2000 years and it originated to Asia. Around 600 BC this vegetable was brought to Europe and it was widely cultivated in Europe until the end of middle Ages. The historical records depict that the ancient Greek people and Romans used to cultivate kale. Finally in 17th century kale was introduced to United States by the European immigrants. Kale is still a common vegetable in Europe, Africa and Asia. The health conscious people in United States give value to this vegetable for it mineral, fiber and vitamin content.

The dark green leafy vegetable with earthy flavor is called kale, which belongs to Acephala cultivarthe of cabbage family. This seasonal vegetable has snatched scientists' attention for its powerful healthy properties. Though kale can be chewed raw but some people prefer cooked one.

Varieties of Kale-
- Redbor Kale
- Siberian Kale
- Ornamental Kale
- Red Russian Kale
- Lacinato or Dino Kale
- Curly leaved or Scots kale

Nutrients in Kale-
- Vitamins- A, B1, B2, B3, B6, C, E and K
- Minerals – Manganese, Copper, Iron, Calcium, Phosphorus, Potassium, Magnesium, Sodium.
- Fiber
- Tryptophan

- Omega-3 fats
- Protein
- Folate
- Folic Acid

Health Benefits:

- **Cancer:** Kale contains glucosinolates, which is believed to have cancer preventive ability. High level of glucosinolates in kale makes it also valuable to treat cancer. Carotonoids and flavonoids are those properties, which give kale the anti-oxidant activity. The 45 different anti-oxidant flavonoids also provide the anti-cancer benefits to kale.

- Being rich in vitamins kale can provide the daily requirements of vitamins into our body.

- Kale is a rich source of vitamin K, which provides the normal bone health and prevents internal blood clotting. It is also studied that vitamin K is helpful to fight against cancer.

- Kale lowers the high cholesterol level and control the cardiovascular health.

- Kale is considered to be the nutritional power house. It can provide the necessary nutrients.

- Sulfur and fiber in kale helps to detoxify liver.

- Kale can prevent asthma, arthritis and autoimmune disorders, as it contains omega-3 fatty acids.

- Di-indolyl-methane in kale works as anti bacterial and anti viral agent.

- Kale is the greatest source of minerals, which can help to regulate and improve the various body functions.

27. QUINOA

Quinoa is a seed from Chenopodium or Goosefoot plant, although it is used as grain in cooking. Quinoa is protein packed seed with mild flavor and it can be used as substitute of rice or couscous. It is highly nutritious and gluten-free seed. Quinoa seed is small-round in shape and it is usually covered with saponin. The seeds should be washed in alkaline solution to remove the cover in order to make it edible. Because of the cover quinoa seeds look blue, orange, blue-black and violet in color but after removing saponin these seeds have the uniform pale-yellow color.

The history of quinoa is 4000 years old and it was native to the Andean region of Peru, Colombia and Bolivia. It was first cultivated by pre-Colombian civilization and it was the staple food until it was replaced by cereals with the Spanish arrival. Around 1200AD quinoa was the main food to the Inca Empire. People first used the leaves and seeds of wild quinoa as the source of food before domestication. In US the quinoa is cultivated in Colorado but most of the supplies are still come from South America.

Quinoa is considered as pseudo grains and it is an enormous source of proteins. Along with the amino acids, it is also a great source of minerals and vitamins. Polyphenols, phytosterols, and flavonoids are other ingredients, which are responsible for the health benefits from this seed. Scientists have found that quinoa seeds also contain vitamin E and Omega-6. With all these active ingredients quinoa seeds still hold the valuable place to all the health conscious people.

Health Benefits

Along with the packed proteins Quinoa seeds supply other health benefits.

- **Iron:** With the iron content quinoa helps the formation of hemoglobin and keeps red blood cells healthy. Iron is the major carrier of oxygen and due to this reason it is also helpful to keep our bran healthy.
- **Fiber:** Quinoa seeds contain more fibers than other grains contain. Fiber helps to reduce constipation and lower the chance of having heart disease. It also controls the cholesterol and glucose level in blood.
- **Antioxidant:** Phytonutrients quercetin and kaempferol in Quinoa seeds give it the anti-oxidant effect and can work as anti-inflammatory.
- **Amino Acids:** Quinoa seeds contain all the nine essential amino acids, which help the process of developing muscle tissues and used by the necessary metabolic enzymes.
- **Quinoa contains Lysine:** Lysine is essential for tissue growth.
- **Riboflavin (B2):** Quinoa contains high level of B2 and this why quinoa helps creating proper energy production in cells and improves metabolism within muscle cells and brain.
- **Magnesium & Manganese:** Quinoa is a rich source of magnesium, which relaxes the blood vessels and alleviates migraines. Magnesium is also helpful, as it promotes healthy blood sugar control and can reduce type-2 diabetes.

  Quinoa also contains manganese, which is considered as an anti-oxidant and it prevents the damage of mitochondria.
- **Blood Pressure:** With the highest level of potassium, quinoa helps to lower the blood pressure. Quinoa also helps to balance the sodium level in blood, which is essential to control the normal blood pressure.
- **Quinoa helps to reduce over weight.**

- The high level of proteins and carbohydrate in quinoa, gives it the ability to regulate the blood sugar.

28. FLAXSEED

Flax is one of the ancient fiber crops and the seeds from it are the huge nutrients source. Flax has been cultivated in ancient Egypt and China. King Charlemagne in 8th century AD made eating flaxseeds as loyal subject, as it has great health benefits. Flaxseeds have been used from thousands of years for medicinal purposes. Ancient Romans, Greeks and Egyptians used to take flaxseed as anti-inflammatory agent and they believed that it could treat gastro-intestinal problems. According to Historia Naturalis (encyclopedia of natural science), the roman naturalist, Pliny the Elder (AD23-79) included thirty uses of flaxseeds. Today the health benefits from flaxseeds are well recognized and cultivated around the world.

Golden flaxseeds and brown flaxseeds are two main types of flaxseeds. Flaxseed along with the flaxseed oil contains alpha-linolenic acid (omega-3 fatty acid), which is considered as more active omega 3 in body. Due to the high fiber content, flaxseed is weighty and thus it is helpful to treat constipation. The American Nutrition Association flaxseed is an excellent source of two types of fatty acids, fibers, minerals and vitamins.

The Flax Council estimates close to 300 new flax-based products were launched in the U.S. and Canada in 2010 alone. Not only has consumer demand for flaxseed grown, agricultural use has also increased. Flaxseed is what's used to feed all those chickens that are laying eggs with higher levels of omega-3 fatty acids. (http://www.webmd.com/diet/features/benefits-of-flaxseed)

Other than the seeds there are two products of flaxseeds available in market- flaxseed oil and ground flaxseed. Flaxseed oil is the fat portion of the seeds and contains high level of omega3 ALA fatty acids, where as ground flaxseeds are rich in fibers and lignans.

Nutritional Properties:

- **Carbohydrtaes-** Dietary fibers, sugar.
- **Proteins-** Thiamine (vitamin-B1), Riboflavin (vitamin-B2), Niacin (vitamin-B3), Pantothenic acid (vitamin-B5), Vitamin-B6, Vitamin-B9, vitamin-C.
- **Minerals-**Iron, Magnesium, Phosphorus, Calcium, Potassium and Zinc.
- **Fat-** saturated, Mono saturated and Poly saturated.

Nutritional facts:

Omega-3 fatty acid: Flaxseeds contain the essential omega-3 fatty acids (linoleic acid, alpha-linolenic acid) and arachidonic acid. These fatty acids help to lower the LDL and higher the HDL. It also prevents the fatal heart attack.

N-3 fatty acid: this fatty acid is helpful to prevent coronary-artery disease and has anti-inflammatory effect. Flaxseed oil is also a source of this fatty acid.

Lignan: It is studied that flaxseed is the highest known concentrations of lignan, which is a major class of phytoestrogens. This phytoestrogens acts like the female hormone estrogen and along with the anti-oxidant compound this phytoestrogens can also fight against cancer.

Fiber: The soluble fibers in flaxseeds dissolve with water and lower the glucose and cholesterol level in blood, as well as maintain the intestine-health. The soluble fibers get a gel like substance with water and this gel promote the bowel movements.

Vitamins: Flaxseeds are the great source of gamma-tocopherol, which is a special compound of vitamin E. This chemical or vitamin E maintains the integrity of cell membrane of mucus membranes.

These seeds are also packed with vitamin B-complex. Regular consumption of flaxseeds during pregnancy can supply the important ingredient folate, which can prevent neural tube defects in the fetus

Health Benefits:

- **Fights against Cancer:** The omega-3 fatty acids (ALA), which can inhibit tumor growth and fight against cancer. It has also been studied that lignans can also prevent breast cancer. "Lignans may help protect against cancer by blocking enzymes that are involved in hormone metabolism and interfering with the growth and spread of tumor cells". (http://www.webmd.com/diet/features/benefits-of-flaxseed). The study, which was presented in American Society of Clinical Oncology, showed that flaxseeds can inhibit the prostate tumor growth and have protective effects on prostate cancer.
- **Prevents Heart disease:** Studies have found that the omega-3 fatty acids, which can look after the cardiovascular health, by normalizing the heart bit and many different mechanisms. Regular consumption of flaxseeds can prevent fatal heart attack. Flaxseeds also lower the LDL cholesterol and increase the HDL cholesterol level.
- Because of the lignans in flaxseeds, diabetes can be prevented by regular use of flaxseeds.
- Flaxseeds prevent hot flashes.
- ALA and lignans in flaxseeds help to protect for inflammation, which can be the cause of various diseases, like- Parkinson's and asthma.
- Flaxseeds protect our skin form radiation.

29. STEEL CUT OATS

This oats are also known as Irish oats or Pinhead oats. The toasted oat grains are cut into small sesame like pieces on steel mill and that is why these oats have got the name 'steel cut oats'. This version of oats have chewy texture and little nuttier than regular oats.

Though steel cut oats go through extra processing steps, they steel have the same amount of nutrients as the primary oats have.

Nutritional Facts:

Protein: Irish oat is the good supply of protein. Protein has some important functions in our body but Irish oats does not have the all nine essential amino acids and that is why it is called incomplete protein.

Minerals & Vitamins: Steel cut oats are the gentle contributor of needed iron in our body. It also has a little amount of calcium which can be a good source of calcium in our body. Other mineral that are present in steel cut oats are zinc, manganese, magnesium, potassium, copper and sodium. It is processed grain but it does lack the content of vitamins.

Fibers & carbohydrates: Steel cut oats can be a regular supplement of carbohydrates. Fiber, which is a kind of carbohydrate, does not break in our body functions. Fiber is needed to lower the heart disease and it improves digestive system.

Health Benefits:

- The Academy of Nutrition and Dietetics have stated that some compounds in steel cut oats can lower the high blood pressure. The soluble fibers in these oats control the blood pressure level. The patients, who are suffering from hypertension, should eat steel cut oats for normalizing the blood pressure.
- The soluble fibers in Irish oats help to prevent heart disease. Regular habit of taking Irish oats can lower the risk of having coronary heart diseases.

- According to American Diabetes Association the low glycemic index in steel cut oats helps to reduce the glucose level in blood and thus it protects from diabetes.
- The low glycemic index is also beneficial in over all weight management activities. Steel cut oats are low in calories, so, it can be a remedy for weight loss.

30. THANK YOU FOR READING!

Thank You so much for reading this book. If this title gave you a ton of value, It would be amazing for you to leave a REVIEW !

THANK YOU FOR DOWNLOADING! IF YOU ENJOYED THIS BOOK AND WOULD LIKE TO READ MORE TITLES FROM MY COLLECTION CLICK THIS LINK

www.ingramcontent.com/pod-product-compliance
Lightning Source LLC
Chambersburg PA
CBHW050414290526
45786CB00003B/1258